Complementary and Alternative Medicine and Psychiatry

Review of Psychiatry Series
John M. Oldham, M.D.
Michelle B. Riba, M.D.
Series Editors

Complementary and Alternative Medicine and Psychiatry

EDITED BY

Philip R. Muskin, M.D.

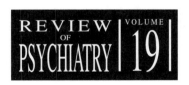

No. 1

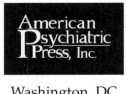

Washington, DC
London, England

Copyright © 2000 American Psychiatric Press, Inc.
04   03   02   01   5   4   3   2

ALL RIGHTS RESERVED
Manufactured in the United States of America on acid-free paper

American Psychiatric Press, Inc.
1400 K Street, NW
Washington, DC 20005
www.appi.org

The correct citation for this book is

Muskin PR (ed.): *Complementary and Alternative Medicine and Psychiatry* (Review of Psychiatry Series, Vol. 19, No. 1; Oldham JM and Riba MB, series eds.). Washington, DC, American Psychiatric Press, 2000

Library of Congress Cataloging-in-Publication Data
Complementary and alternative medicine and psychiatry /
    edited by Philip R. Muskin
        p. ; cm. — (Review of psychiatry ; v. 19, no. 1)
    Includes bibliographical references and index.
    ISBN 0-88048-174-9 (alk. paper)
    1. Alternative medicine. 2. Psychiatry. I. Muskin, Philip R. II. Review of Psychiatry series ; v. 19, 1.
        [DNLM: 1. Alternative Medicine. 2. Psychiatry—methods.
    3. Psychotherapy—methods.
    WB 890 C7366 2000]
    R733.C6528 2000
    615.5—dc21

British Library Cataloguing in Publication Data
A CIP record is available from the British Library.

Review of Psychiatry Series ISSN 1041-5882

Contents

Chapter 5

Complementary Medicine: Implications Toward Medical Treatment and the Patient–Physician Relationship

Catherine C. Crone, M.D.

Thomas N. Wise, M.D.

Philip R. Muskin, M.D.

Contributors

Ina Becker, M.D., Ph.D.
Assistant Director, Center for Meditation and Healing, Columbia University; Assistant Professor of Clinical Psychiatry, Columbia University College of Physicians & Surgeons, New York, New York

Richard P. Brown, M.D.
Associate Professor of Clinical Psychiatry, Columbia University College of Physicians & Surgeons, New York, New York

Catherine C. Crone, M.D.
Director, Consultation-Liaison Psychiatry Fellowship, Department of Psychiatry, Inova Fairfax Hospital/Georgetown University, Falls Church, Virginia; Assistant Clinical Professor, Department of Psychiatry, Georgetown University Medical Center, Washington, DC

Patricia L. Gerbarg, M.D.
Assistant Clinical Professor of Psychiatry, New York Medical College, New York, New York

Joseph Loizzo, M.D., M.Phil.
Founder and Director, Clinical Center for Meditation and Healing, Columbia-Presbyterian Eastside; Assistant Professor of Clinical Psychiatry, Columbia University College of Physicians & Surgeons; Presidential Fellow in Indo-Tibetan Studies, Columbia University Graduate School of Arts and Sciences, New York, New York

Philip R. Muskin, M.D.
Chief, Consultation-Liaison Psychiatry, Columbia-Presbyterian Medical Center; Associate Professor of Clinical Psychiatry, Columbia University College of Physicians & Surgeons; and Faculty, Columbia University Psychoanalytic Center for Training and Research, New York, New York

John M. Oldham, M.D.
Director, New York State Psychiatric Institute; Dollard Professor and Acting Chairman, Department of Psychiatry, Columbia University College of Physicians and Surgeons, New York, New York

Francine Rainone, D.O.

Department of Family Medicine, Department of Pain Medicine and Palliative Care, Coordinator or Curriculum in Complementary and Alternative Medicine, Director of Continuing Medical Education in Complementary and Alternative Medicine, and Residency Program in Urban Family Health, Beth Israel Medical Center; Assistant Professor of Family Medicine, Albert Einstein College of Medicine, New York, New York

Michelle B. Riba, M.D.

Clinical Associate Professor of Psychiatry and Associate Chair for Education and Academic Affairs, Department of Psychiatry, University of Michigan Health System, Ann Arbor, Michigan

Thomas N. Wise, M.D.

Chairman, Department of Psychiatry, Inova Fairfax Hospital, Falls Church, Virginia; Vice Chairman and Professor, Department of Psychiatry, Georgetown University Medical Center, Washington, DC; Professor, Department of Psychiatry, Johns Hopkins University School of Medicine, Baltimore, Maryland

Introduction to the Review of Psychiatry Series

John M. Oldham, M.D.
Michelle B. Riba, M.D., Series Editors

2000 REVIEW OF PSYCHIATRY SERIES TITLES

- *Learning Disabilities: Implications for Psychiatric Treatment*
  EDITED BY LAURENCE L. GREENHILL, M.D.
- *Psychotherapy for Personality Disorders*
  EDITED BY JOHN G. GUNDERSON, M.D., AND GLEN O. GABBARD, M.D.
- *Ethnicity and Psychopharmacology*
  EDITED BY PEDRO RUIZ, M.D.
- *Complementary and Alternative Medicine and Psychiatry*
  EDITED BY PHILIP R. MUSKIN, M.D.
- *Pain: What Psychiatrists Need to Know*
  EDITED BY MARY JANE MASSIE, M.D.

The advances in knowledge in the field of psychiatry and the neurosciences in the last century can easily be described as breathtaking. As we embark on a new century and a new millennium, we felt that it would be appropriate for the 2000 Review of Psychiatry Series monographs to take stock of the state of that knowledge at the interface between normality and pathology. Although there may be nothing new under the sun, we are learning more about not-so-new things, such as how we grow and develop; who we are; how to differentiate between just being different from one another and being ill; how to recognize, treat, and perhaps prevent illness; how to identify our unique vulnerabilities; and how to deal with the inevitable stress and pain that await each of us.

In the early years of life, for example, how can we tell whether a particular child is just rowdier, less intelligent, or more adventuresome than another child—or is, instead, a child with a learning or behavior disorder? Clearly, the distinction is crucial, because newer and better treatments that now exist for early-onset disorders can smooth the path and enhance the chances for a solid future for children with such disorders. Yet, inappropriately labeling and treating a rambunctious but normal child can create problems rather than solve them. Greenhill and colleagues guide us through these waters, illustrating that a highly sophisticated methodology has been developed to make this distinction with accuracy, and that effective treatments and interventions are now at hand.

Once we have successfully navigated our way into early adulthood, we are supposed to have a pretty good idea (so the advice books say) of who we are. Of course, this stage of development does not come easy, nor at the same time, for all. Again, a challenge presents itself—that is, to differentiate between widely disparate varieties of temperament and character and when extremes of personality traits and styles should be recognized as disorders. And even when traits are so extreme that little dispute exists that a disorder is present, does that disorder represent who the person is, or is it something the individual either inherited or developed and might be able to overcome? In the fifth century B.C., Hippocrates described different personality types that he proposed were correlated with specific "body humors"; this ancient principle remains quite relevant, though the body humors of today are neurotransmitters. How low CNS serotonin levels need to be, for example, to produce disordered impulsivity is still being determined, yet new symptom-targeted treatment of such conditions with SSRIs is now well accepted. What has been at risk as the neurobiology of personality disorders has become increasingly understood is the continued recognition of the importance of psychosocial treatments for these disorders. Gunderson and Gabbard and their colleagues review the surprisingly robust evidence for the effectiveness of these approaches, including new uses and types of cognitive-behavioral and psychoeducational methods.

It is not just differences in personality that distinguish us from one another. Particularly in our new world of global communication and population migration, ethnic and cultural differences are more often part of life in our own neighborhoods than just exotic and unfamiliar aspects of faraway lands. Despite great strides overcoming fears and prejudices, much work remains to be done. At the same time, we must learn more about ways that we are different (not better or worse) genetically and biologically, because uninformed ignorance of these differences leads to unacceptable risks. Ruiz and colleagues carefully present what we now know and do not know about ethnicity and its effects on pharmacokinetics and pharmacodynamics.

An explosion of interest in and information about wellness—not just illness—surrounds us. How to achieve and sustain a healthy lifestyle, how to enhance successful aging, and how to benefit from "natural" remedies saturate the media. Ironically, although this seems to be a new phenomenon, the principles of complementary or alternative medicine are ancient. Some of our oldest and most widely used medications are derived from plants and herbs, and Eastern medicine has for centuries relied on concepts of harmony, relaxation, and meditation. Again, as the world shrinks, we are obligated to be open to ideas that may be new to us but not to others and to carefully evaluate their utility. Muskin and colleagues present a careful analysis of the most familiar and important components of complementary and alternative medicine, presenting a substantial database of information, along with tutorials on non-Western (hence nontraditional to us) concepts and beliefs.

Like it or not, life presents us with stress and pain. Pain management has not typically figured into mainstream psychiatric training or practice (with the exception of consultation-liaison psychiatry), yet it figures prominently in the lives of us all. Massie and colleagues provide us with a primer on what psychiatrists should know about the subject, and there is a great deal indeed that we should know.

Many other interfaces exist between psychiatry as a field of medicine, defining and treating psychiatric illnesses, and the rest of medicine—and between psychiatry and the many paths of the life cycle. These considerations are, we believe, among our top priorities as we begin the new millennium, and these volumes provide an in-depth review of some of the most important ones.

Introduction:
Herbs and Hermeneutics

Philip R. Muskin, M.D.

"There are more things in heaven and earth, Horatio, than are
dreamt of in your philosophy"

Hamlet Act 1, scene 5

What is alternative medicine? Attempts to define what is conventional and what is not conventional introduce a bias, no matter who the arbiter is who sets up the definitions (Table 1). Many alternative therapies pre-date conventional medicine by hundreds or thousands of years. Some are quite well known, others seem mysterious or strange, and some pose serious risks (Murray and Rubel 1992). Many of us use unconventional therapies acquired from grandparents, parents, or friends (chicken soup is perhaps the most famous) in our personal lives without a second thought. In some circles alternative medicine is completely dismissed (Funtanarosa and Lundberg 1998). Yet those who contend that alternative therapies have no value may be guilty of failing to adhere to one of the core aphorisms of medicine, that is, "Never say never." Special diets, ritualistic practices, gleaning information about people in unconventional ways, healing based on energy fields or aromas, and other unusual methods may cause some physicians to warn patients away from complementary and alternative medicine (CAM). Is it pure science that supports our faith in "allopathic" medicine, or do the character traits that many physicians possess influence our rejection of what seems to be less well substantiated therapies (Gabbard 1985)?

What differentiates CAM approaches from conventional, or allopathic, medicine is the idea of using the individual's own resources as well as energy within and outside of the person in order to maintain wellness. There is a belief that the body can heal itself, using energy mobilized by external manipulations. The central focus is the individual, not the doctor or the treatment. The unique

Table 1. Types of complementary and alternative medicine

Body	Mind	Spirit
Acupuncture	Adlerian analysis	Absent healing
Aikido	Alexandrian analysis	Catholic healers
Air therapy	Astrology	Edgar Cayce
Alexander method	Bach's flower remedies	Christian Science
Apple cider vinegar and honey (D. D. Jarvis, M.D.)	Bioenergetics	Contact healing
Ayurvedic medicine	Biofeedback training	Eckankar
Biochemics	Direct decision therapy	Enlightened healing
Bioelectromagnetics	Ericksonian analysis	Evangelistic healing
Chinese remedial therapy	est	Gurdjieff
Chiropody	Existent analysis	Meditation
Chiropractic	Frommian analysis	Mind power
Color therapy	Gestalt therapy	Palmistry
Coué's autosuggestion	Graphology	Paradox therapy
Dance therapy	Hornevian therapy	Pecci-Hoffman therapy
Earth therapy	Imagery	Primal therapy
Feldenkrais	Jungian analysis	Radiesthesia
Gravitonics	Logotherapy (Victor Frankl)	Rankian therapy
Herbalism	Maslovian analysis	Rational therapy
Homeopathy	Mensendick system	Reichian therapy
Hypnosis	Moxibustion	Reikian analysis
Ionization	Music therapy	Scientology
Iriodology	Naprapathy	Spiritualists
Japanese massage	Naturopathy	Sullivanian analysis
Kneipp's water therapy	Osteopathy	Transactional analysis
Lakhovsky oscillatory coils	Phrenology	Yoga
Lotte Berk method	Phrenosophical spiritual healing	Zen
Massage	Polarity therapy	
Sleep therapy	Radiesthesia	
Spiritual healing	Reich's orgonic therapy	
Structural integration (Rolfing)	Rikli's sunshine cure	
Tai chi ch'uan	Sauna	
Tantric medicine	Sex therapy	
Unani medicine	Shiatsu massage	

Table 1. Types of complementary and alternative medicine *(continued)*

Body	Mind	Spirit
Vitamin therapy	Visualization	
Yoga		
Zen macrobiotics		

Source. LaPatra 1978

quality of the whole person in alternative therapies makes the concepts of standardization, quantification, generalization, and normalization problematic for both research and clinical activity in comparison with conventional medicine. In allopathic medicine, the treatment acts on the person, who plays no active role beyond cooperation with the treatment regimen; the knowledge rests with the doctor. In alternative medicine, the knowledge and beliefs are shared by patients and practitioners with a focus on what is unique about the patient and on his or her role in self-healing. In CAM, natural products, plants, and nutrients all play an important role, because the body exists in an environment from which it is designed to obtain energy, stay healthy, and get well.

When we look back at some of the claims made by proponents of certain therapies, they may seem absurd, even frightening. Yet not all of the ideas are unworthy of consideration. For example, in 1839 Sylvester Graham, a Presbyterian minister, espoused the value of dietary measures for good health in two volumes entitled *Lectures on the Science of Life.* Graham blamed American dyspepsia on fried meat, alcohol, eating too fast, and the use of "unnatural" refined wheat flour. He urged people to eat fruits, vegetables, and unsifted whole wheat flour (*graham* flour) in bread that is slightly stale and to chew thoroughly to promote good digestion, prevent alcoholism, and diminish the sex urge. Graham's teaching came from his religious beliefs that all pleasurable sensation was Satanic in origin and that immoral behavior resulted in poor health. Adherents of Graham's philosophy did not eat meat, drank a lot of water, bathed regularly, and believed corsets and neckties were bad for them—not a particularly bad way to live. In addition, graham flour was an important ingredient in the graham crackers they ate. In our modern world, would we not be worse off without the pleasure of a "s'more"(*graham* cracker, roasted marshmallow, and chocolate) at a campfire cookout?

When we question the efficacy of a dose of medication seemingly too small to have a clinical effect, we label it as a *homeopathic* dose. Homeopathy derives from a principle voiced by Hippocrates in 400 B.C., *similia similibus curantur*, or "like cures like." Samuel Hahnemann founded homeopathy in 1796, and it once enjoyed great worldwide popularity. A central principle of homeopathy is that a person with an illness can be cured by a substance that causes symptoms similar to that illness. Homeopaths contend that minuscule quantities of the substance will bring out the body's natural healing mechanisms and thus dilute the material until only infinitesimal quantities are left in solution. Critics of homeopathy are both new and old. In 1999, *The Medical Letter* concluded "there is no good reason to use" homeopathic products ("Homeopathic products" 1999). One hundred fifty-seven years earlier, Oliver Wendell Holmes delivered two lectures to the Boston Society for the Diffusion of Useful Knowledge entitled, "Homeopathy and Its Kindred Delusions." He commented, "I think it fair to conclude that the catalogues of symptoms attributed in Homeopathic works to the influence of various drugs upon healthy persons are not entitled to any confidence" (Holmes 1985). If everyone had followed Holmes regarding homeopathic principles, then no one would have taken the letter by Reverend Edmund Stone to the Royal College of Physicians seriously. He described "an account of the success of the bark of the willow in the cure of agues" (Insel 1996). Because willow grows in swamps where agues (fevers) are known to occur, Reverend Stone thought that willow would have curative powers for fevers. In 1829, salicin was isolated from willow bark. Felix Hoffman, a chemist with the Bayer Corporation, synthesized acetylsalicylic acid in the later part of the 1800s. In 1905 this was marketed by Bayer as *aspirin*, a name derived from *Spiraea*, a plant from which salicylic acid was prepared. Thus the discovery of aspirin, one of the wonder drugs of the twentieth century, was directly related to homeopathic principles, and the substance was derived from a botanical product in use for hundreds of years by native peoples.

It is difficult not to throw out the "baby" of efficacious alternative treatments with the "bath water" of the failure to substantiate many of the claims regarding alternative therapies. Many important treatments derive from natural substances, including Taxol and several other antineoplastics. Natural-product drugs comprise 34% of the 25 best-selling drugs (Service 1999). Penicillin started out as a mold. The leaves of the foxglove plant (*Digitalis purpurea*) contain digitoxin and were used more than 300 years ago for the treatment of dropsy (edema related to congestive heart failure). If we dismiss the value of the natural world, other effective treatments—both biological and psychological—might not be discovered. Ten years ago there was much excitement about finding new treatments from natural sources. The cost of finding, isolating, purifying, and testing natural substances is so high that some companies have abandoned the search and instead use combinational chemistry to synthesize thousands of compounds and then screen them for potential drugs (Service 1999). Many companies, however, continue the search for natural products, using improved technology to purify and analyze compounds or isolating natural products from microorganisms (Service 1999). Those who are open minded toward natural products may believe in two widely held notions, that *natural is safer* and that *natural is better* than conventional treatments. Neither of these approaches is completely true.

Natural is **not** always safer. Botanical products are not subject to the stringent regulations of the U.S. Food and Drug Administration. Although claims may be made in advertisements or by celebrities, these products are not medications but are dietary supplements. The consumer may or may not be getting what he or she expects in the preparation. Botanical dietary supplements are regulated under the Dietary Supplement Health and Education Act of 1994, which does not require that the substance be shown to be safe and effective for the indication (Slifman et al. 1998). Serious and potentially lethal contamination of botanical supplements is possible and has occurred (Slifman et al. 1998). MuTong, a Chinese herbal tea used for eczema, has caused renal failure requiring kidney transplant (Lord et al. 1999). This condition apparently results from failure to accurately pick the plant from which the tea is prepared. As those with a garden know well, in some years a particular plant may grow well, but not every year. Thus the herbal preparation may contain none, some, or too much of the ingredient that yields the desired therapeutic effect. Preparations found in health food stores may contain little of the "active" substance (Davidson 1999). Although some adverse herb–drug reactions have been described, interactions between "natural" products and medications are unknown for the most part, leading to potentially adverse reactions (Yager 1999). Some patients may tell their physicians of their use of alternative therapies, but not 100% of patients. Herbs have the potential to cause adverse interactions with anesthesia (Nagourney 1999), particularly problematic if the physician is unaware of the patient's use of an herbal preparation. *Ginkgo biloba* and *Allium sativum* (garlic) may both result in bleeding if taken along with anticoagulants (Brody 1999, Calvo 1999). *Hypericum perforatum* (St. John's wort), *Ginkgo biloba*, and *Echinacea purpurea* have been shown to be damaging to reproductive cells in animal studies (Ondrizek et al. 1999). St. John's wort may induce hepatic enzymes to metabolize other drugs such as indinavir more quickly (Piscitelli et al. 2000). This could reduce the effectiveness of medications used to treat AIDS or prevent transplant rejection. These concerns are particularly important when St. John's wort is used as an alternative to antidepressant treatment without medical supervision and when ginkgo is recommended as adjunctive therapy for patients experiencing sexual dysfunction secondary to treatment with traditional antidepressants (Cohen and Bartlik 1998). Ephedra (*ma huang*), used as a stimulant and decongestant, has been linked to over 38 deaths ("Herbal Rx" 1999). Patients taking psychiatric drugs may add on alternative therapies that produce toxicity, benefit, or confuse both patient and physician as to which substance was the therapeutic agent (Yager et al. 1999). There is little to support the notion of natural substances carrying a greater degree of safety than pharmaceutical products. If the substances are effective, they are drugs in a natural form. All drugs have the potential to cause harm.

Alternative therapies are not new and in using them we have now gone full circle back to more primitive forms of treatment.

Alternative therapies have always been there, and people have always used them. The concept of a vital energy is found in *homeopathy* (spiritual vital force), *chiropractic* (innate energy), *psychic healing* (auric, psionic), *acupuncture* (*qi*), *ayurvedic medicine* (*prana*), or *naturopathy* (*vis medicatrix naturae*) (Kaptchuk 1996). There is a belief in forces, invisible but powerful, that exert an effect on us all and must be used to maintain wellness and restore health. If the concept of vitalism is traced from its Aristotelian and Asian roots, the path leads through Mesmer's animal magnetism, Rhine's parapsychology, von Reichenbach's odic force of crystal healing, and Quimby's Mind Cure. In Mind Cure, disease is thought to be the product of wrong thinking. Meditation, relaxation, and deep breathing help autosuggestion that would result in cure. One of Quimby's students (and patients) was Mary Baker Eddy, who established Christian Science. She espoused the belief that all illness is illusion.

D. D. Palmer was an American mesmeric healer who used hand passes and magnetic spine rubs. In 1895 he had the insight that "putting down your hands"—that is, making mechanical adjustments—worked better than the "laying on of hands." He thus invented chiropractic medicine with the theory that disease derives from too much or too little energy. Spinal alignment frees the nerves to allow innate energy to produce healing. Today, chiropractic medicine is licensed in all 50 states.

Alternative medicine includes another energy that is not connected to either mesmerism or vitalist notions, that is, the healing force of nature or *vis medicatrix naturae* put forward by William Cullen in 1772. This healing energy of nature formed the foundation of the herbalist movement, although herbs had been used for hundreds of years or more by native peoples. The movement became popular in the United States in the 1700s and 1800s with the creation of herbalist medical schools but waned after the last herbal medical school closed in 1939. The herbalist approach also became popular in Europe, where it remains strong even today.

Asian concepts of vital energy (*qi*), part of acupuncture and other disciplines, became popular in the 1960s in the United States. Animate and inanimate matter is said to possess qi. With these new concepts come new types of massage, such as shiatsu; new concepts of energy, such as reiki johrei; and new forms of meditation.

The concept of vital energy went in many directions. In 1843 James Braid postulated that mesmerism had its effects via a mental force that he named *hypnosis*. This notion was taken up and explored by Charcot and Bernheim, with whom Freud studied. Freud used hypnosis in his early work, and this formed the foundation for his psychoanalytic theory, which informed the psychotherapies that use psychodynamic concepts. The fusion of the concepts of hypnosis, autogenic training (specific self-instructions to relax), and guided imagery with the work of Pavlov, Watson, and Thorndike led to the creation of biofeedback. *Biofeedback* uses the person's ability to self-train and control internal physiologic responses in order to treat illness and maintain wellness. These concepts led Benson to conceptualize the Relaxation Response. In the 1920s the term *holistic medicine* was coined by J. C. Smuts, a South African statesman. The term was both antivitalist and antimechanistic. This antireductionist approach contends that the whole of the organism cannot be explained by its parts. Later antireductionists in biomedicine such as Cannon, Seyle, Dunbar, and Engels focused on people's predispositions, psychosocial factors, and homeostasis. From an ancient belief in the vital energy of all things, a concept that might be rejected as unscientific and unprovable, we arrive at concepts that are part of our everyday work. In tracing the history of vital energy and alternative medicine it becomes difficult to know what is alternative to what.

Is natural better? This is a question of perspective, because there is no scientific evidence to support this belief. A meta-analysis of trials of St. John's wort indicated that it is more effective than placebo for mild to moderate depression (Gaster et al. 2000; Linde et al. 1996). There have been many critiques of this literature, particularly questioning the high placebo response rate and the low doses of comparison antidepressants used. Trials comparing St. John's wort with traditional antidepressants in the United States are under way. Early on in the history of the selective serotonin reuptake inhibitors (SSRIs)—as recently as 1989—people asked similar questions about this new class of drugs. If a patient uses an alternative therapy and recovers, and this treatment is psychologically more acceptable than a conventional treatment that the person would not have undertaken, how do we then define better? What defines natural? Any treatment that exerts an effect psychologically, whether good or bad, must do so via the brain. Wherever the mind is, one must first go through the brain to get to the mind. From a narrow perspective, therapies that employ talk as the central element are all "natural," whatever the theory that informs the therapy, because humankind has sought to understand itself for as long as there has been recorded history. Successful therapy employing talk has been shown to change the functioning of the brain, as demonstrated by positron-emission tomography (PET) scans (Schwartz et al. 1996). If talk is natural but works to change the brain, there is a blurring of the distinction between therapies that conventional physicians might call alternative and those they view as traditional. Patients, however, seem to take to these alternative therapies much more readily than do some physicians.

Some of the popularity of these therapies comes from their reputation; we have heard about the benefits, know of someone who has benefited, or have personally experienced a benefit from some alternative treatment. In some cases the treatment actually has exerted a therapeutic effect, even if the mechanism is unknown. St. John's wort, now under consideration as an antidepressant, is also a folk remedy for skin injuries and burns. Highly purified extracts of *Hypericum perforatum* demonstrate antibacterial properties (Schempp et al. 1999). In preantibiotic times, an extract of St. John's wort might well have prevented an infection when applied to burns or wounds. Because no treatment, conventional or alternative, works 100% of the time, even occasional successes build the reputation of efficacy. On the other hand, the plural of anecdote is not data.

Another factor influencing the positive reputation of alternative therapies is the placebo effect. *Placebo,* or "I shall please," was defined in 1785 as a "commonplace method or medicine" (Straus and von Ammon Cavanaugh 1996). We attribute the efficacy of a treatment that lacks a known mechanism or theory of action to beliefs that the culture chooses to overlook (Hahn 1985). The power of placebo cannot be ignored, however, although we might wish that it remain confined to alternative treatments. There is the possibility of a placebo response as a minor or major effect even when an "active" treatment is undertaken. Placebo responders occur in every drug trial. Even in a study of lowering cholesterol, patients in the placebo group had a lower mortality rate as long as they were compliant with the placebo (Coronary Drug Project Group 1980). When subjects have experience with a substance (in this instance alcohol), their *belief* that they have received the active substance equals the effect of the active substance itself (Himie et al. 1999). The expectations of patient and doctor regarding a treatment influence the outcome, positively and negatively (Smith and Thompson 1993). *Nocebo*, or "I shall harm," responses also occur and are well-known in drug trials in patients receiving active and placebo treatments.

The power of the mind must always be respected in its control over both psyche and soma. Thus, in pharmacologic and non-pharmacologic therapies, whether alternative or conventional, the patient's, practitioner's, family's, and culture's emotions and fantasies influence the outcome. A recent meta-analysis of antidepressants suggested that the placebo response accounts for 75% of the response in drug trials (Kirsch and Sapirstein 1998). Although this controversial critique raises important questions, most physicians who use medications contend that there are pharmacologic effects that have produced great benefit for patients. How powerful can the mind be? Our clinical experience exposes us to the devastating power of the mind in psychiatric disorders. Some would discount therapies that rely on the alteration of energy, mediation, or spirituality. How can we explain the prolonged survival of women with cancer who participate in supportive group therapy? (See Fawzy et al. 1993; Spiegel et al. 1989.) Seemingly impossible achievements can occur with desire and practice. To use an example outside of the alternative medicine field: studies of karate demonstrated that a well-trained karateka (practitioner of karate) kicks at speeds of greater than 21,000 mph (Feld et al. 1979). The power generated in a karate punch is equivalent to the energy necessary to lift a 1-ton weight several inches off the floor (Feld et al. 1979). Is it impossible that a person's focus of internal resources could not be used to exert a healing effect, even if we do not understand the mechanism?

Data from a telephone survey of 2,055 adults in 1997 formed the basis of an estimate that $21.2 billion to $32.7 billion are spent annually on alternative therapies in the United States, most of which is out of pocket (Eisenberg et al. 1998). This 1997 survey found a 45% increase in use from a 1990 study (Eisenberg et al. 1993). Only 38.5% of the participants discussed their use of alternative therapy with their medical doctor, and 46.5% of people used CAM for a medical condition without supervision from either a medical doctor or a practitioner of alternative therapy. It is easy to dismiss these data as insignificant for conditions such as sprains/strains, headaches, or fatigue. But people also treated their hypertension, allergies, lung problems, depression, and anxiety with alternative therapies. Some of these treatments may be efficacious, whereas others may work via the power of the placebo effect. How comfortable are we as health professionals to have no idea where the therapeutic effect comes from? How many of these people might have been effectively treated by conventional therapies but remained untreated because they used ineffective CAM therapies?

A recent study indicated that 28% of women who have had surgery for breast cancer use CAM therapies (Burstein et al. 1999). Of these women, 71% informed their doctors of their CAM use. These therapies did not replace the use of conventional treatments, suggesting that these women used the therapies as complementary rather than alternative. Those women who used CAM therapies had the greatest degree of psychologic distress (measured by more depression, lower levels of sexual satisfaction, increased fear of disease recurrence, and a greater frequency and severity of somatic symptoms). The study suggests that some patients use CAM therapies to reduce their psychologic distress rather than replace conventional treatments in which they had no faith. It indicates that the problem is not the use of the therapies, but the failure of the physicians to recognize and address the patient's emotional distress (Holland 1999).

We might then speculate about the meaning of the widespread use of alternative medicine. One obvious meaning is the person's attempt to gain mastery over a body and/or mind that is being experienced as out of control. Natural or alternative therapies carry none of the stigma associated with conventional treatment, particularly psychiatric treatment. Many patients tell no one of their use of alternative therapy, suggesting that the use of these approaches is a private way to reestablish an emotional homeostasis. If the approach to the problem is "natural," then the person can deny that there is anything wrong. This belief is fueled by denial, and thus the choice of alternative medicine is founded on fear. Denial can play a powerful role in the maladaptive response to physical illness (Muskin et al. 1998; Strauss et al. 1990). Some people reject the structure of allopathic medicine, mistrust the institution of the hospital, and dislike the authority of the doctor. The centrality of the patient's individuality, his or her role in the healing process, and the shared knowledge and beliefs with the alternative medicine practitioner create an atmosphere that these people can accept. This atmosphere could be created within conventional medicine, but it is often missing. Increasing physicians' communication skills is a major step in this direction (Roter and Hall 1993). Other patients, such as those in the Burstein et al. (1999) study mentioned earlier, add unproved but potentially therapeutic approaches to their conventional therapies out of fear that not all that can be done for them will be accomplished through traditional medicine. In some cases, perhaps many, the use of alternative medicine is a signal that the patient feels frightened and helpless but is unable to communicate these concerns to the physician. If we can recognize the metaphor and respond to the patient appropriately, this communication could foster a more supportive and therapeutic patient–physician relationship.

This volume focuses on several areas within CAM. The authors are all physicians who live in the worlds of both allopathic and alternative medicine. No book could be exhaustive, because there is too much to know. Our hope is to provide practitioners with a basic knowledge so that they may respond to patients' questions, guide patients regarding therapies, and open their minds. In the chapter by Drs. Brown and Gerbarg you will find a thorough review of herbals and nutrients for treatment of a variety of conditions, both medical and psychiatric. In this and other chapters we have included many original sources for those who wish to read the studies themselves. Dr. Rainone's chapter on acupuncture presents illness and treatment from the perspective of someone who is trained in both allopathic medicine and Chinese medicine. The chapter on yoga by Dr. Becker reviews both the concepts that inform yoga practice and how yoga can be added to the conventional practice of psychiatry. In Dr. Loizzo's chapter on mediation, the complexity of meditative practice and its role for the psychiatrist are carefully delineated. Finally, Drs. Crone and Wise review the practical concomitants of CAM use by patients with medical illness.

As you read these chapters consider the following actual case:

> A man, aged 45 years, is admitted with end-stage heart disease awaiting a cardiac transplant. He requires a left ventricular assist device (LVAD) along with several medications for his heart to keep him alive. Without the medications and the LVAD he will surely die. The passive role is intolerable for him, and he is non-compliant with his diet and medications. The staff find him frightening because he is aggressive. The psychiatric consultant engages this patient in a discussion of his concerns, fears, and behavior. The psychiatrist uses a psychodynamic life narrative to explain to this man how he comes to this point in his life, at this time, enabling him to understand himself and thus find it easier to comply with the treatment. He is better able to tolerate his situation and wait for a heart transplant. (Viederman and Perry 1980)

Without the psychotherapy this man will surely die. But without the pharmacotherapy and mechanical device this man will also die. Which is the *complementary* therapy to the one keeping him alive?

Resources on the Internet

Healthwwweb: *www.HealthWWWeb.com*

Columbia University Rosenthal Center for Alternative/Complementary Medicine: *cpmcnet.columbia.edu/dept/rosenthal/*

Columbia University Rosenthal Center directory of databases: *cpmcnet.columbia.edu/dept/rosenthal/Databases.html*

National Center for Complementary and Alternative Medicine: *altmed.od.nih.gov/nccam*

Alternative and complementary medicine topics: *www.people. virginia.edu/~pjb3s/Complementary_Practices.html*

References

Brody JE: Americans gamble on herbs as medicine. New York Times, February 9, 1999, p F1

Burstein HJ, Gelber S, Guadagnoli E, et al: Use of alternative medicine by women with early-stage breast cancer. N Engl J Med 340:1733–1739, 1999

Calvo T: Natural remedies: what's safe, what's risky? McCall's, August 1999, pp 73–79

Cohen AJ, Bartlik B: Ginkgo biloba for antidepressant-induced sexual dysfunction. J Sex Marital Ther 24:139–143, 1998

Coronary Drug Project Group: Influence of adherence to treatment and response of cholesterol on mortality in the coronary drug project. N Engl J Med 303:1038–1041, 1980

Davidson JRT: St. John's wort: should we be using it for depression? Research advances in medicine, Paper presented at the annual meeting of the American Psychiatric Association, Washington, DC, May 1999

Eisenberg DM, Kessier RC, Foster C, et al: Unconventional medicine in the United States: prevalence, costs, and patterns of use. N Engl J Med 328:246–252, 1993

Eisenberg DM, Davis RB, Ettner SL: Trends in alternative medicine use in the United States, 1990–1997: results of a follow-up national survey. JAMA 280:1569–1575, 1998

Fawzy FI, Fawzy NW, Hyun CS, et al: Malignant melanoma: effects of an early structured psychiatric intervention, coping, and affective state on recurrence and survival 6 years later. Arch Gen Psychiatry 50:681–689, 1993

Feld MS, McNair RE, Wilk SR: The physics of karate. Sci Am 240:150–158, 1979

Funtanarosa PB, Lundberg GD: Alternative medicine meets science. JAMA 280:1618–1619, 1998

Gabbard GO: The role of compulsiveness in the normal physician. JAMA 254:2926–2929, 1985

Gaster B, Holroyd J: St. John's wort for depression. Arch Intern Med 160:152–156, 2000

Hahn RA: A sociocultural model of illness and healing, in Placebo: Theory, Research, and Mechanisms. Edited by White L, Tursky B, Schwartz G. New York, Guilford, 1985, pp 167–195

Herbal Rx: the promise and the pitfalls. Consumer Reports 64:44–48, 1999

Himie JA, Abelson JL, Haghightgou H, et al: Effect of alcohol on social phobic anxiety. Am J Psychiatry 156:1237–1243, 1999

Holland J: Use of alternative medicine: a marker for distress? N Engl J Med 340:758–759, 1999

Holmes OW: Homeopathy, in Examining Holistic Medicine. Edited by Stalker D, Glymour C. Buffalo, NY, Prometheus Books, 1985, pp 221–243

Homepathic products. Med Lett Drugs Ther 41:20–21, 1999

Insel PA: Analgesic-antipyretic and anti-inflammatory agents and drugs employed in the treatment of gout, in Goodman & Gilman's The Pharmacological Basis of Therapeutics, 9th Edition. Edited by Hardman JG, Limbird LE, Molinoff PB, et al. New York, McGraw-Hill, 1996, pp 617–658

Kaptchuk TJ: Historical context of the concept of vitalism in complementary and alternative medicine, in Fundamentals of Complementary and Alternative Medicine. Edited by Micozzi MS. New York, Churchill Livingstone, 1996, pp 35–48

Kirsch I, Sapirstein G: Listening to Prozac but hearing placebo: a meta-analysis of antidepressant medication. Prevention & Treatment (serial online) 1998. Available at http://www.journals.apa.org/prevention/volume1/pre0010002a.html, Accessed June 14, 1999

LaPatra J: Healing: The Coming Revolution in Holistic Medicine. New York, McGraw-Hill, 1978, pp 92–120

Linde K, Ramirez G, Mulrow CD, et al: St John's wort for depression: an overview and meta-analysis of randomised clinical trials. BMJ 313:253–258, 1996

Lord GM, Tagore R, Cook T, et al: Nephropathy caused by Chinese herbs in the UK. Lancet 354:481–482, 1999

Murray RH, Rubel AJ: Physicians and healers—unwitting partners in health care. N Engl J Med 326:61–64, 1992

Muskin PR, Feldhammer T, Gelfand JL, et al: Maladaptive denial of physical illness: a useful new "diagnosis." Int J Psychiatry Med 28:503–517, 1998

Nagourney E: A warning not to mix surgery and herbs. New York Times, July 6, 1999, p F5

Ondrizek RR, Chan PJ, Patton WC, et al: An alternative medicine study of herbal effects on the penetration of zona-free hamster oocytes and the integrity of sperm deoxyribonucleic acid. Fertil Steril 71:517–522, 1999

Piscitelli SC, Burstein AH, Chaitt D, et al: Indinavir concentrations and St. John's wort. Lancet 355:547–548, 2000

Roter DL, Hall JA: Doctors Talking with Patients/Patients Talking with Doctors. Westport, CT, Auburn House, 1993

Schempp CM, Pelz K, Wittmer A, et al: Antibacterial activity of hyperforin from St. John's wort, against multiresistant *Staphylococcus aureus* and gram-positive bacteria. Lancet 353:2129, 1999

Schwartz JM, Stoessel PW, Baxter LR, et al: Systematic changes in cerebral glucose metabolic rate after successful behavior modification treatment of obsessive-compulsive disorder. Arch Gen Psychiatry 53:109–113, 1996

Service RF: Drug industry looks to the lab instead of rainforest and reef. Science 285:186, 1999

Slifman NR, Obermeyer WR, Musser SM, et al: Contamination of botanical dietary supplements by *Digitalis lanata*. N Engl J Med 339:806–811, 1998

Smith TC, Thompson TL: The inherent, powerful therapeutic value of a good physician-patient relationship. Psychosomatics 3:166–170, 1993

Spiegel D, Bloom JR, Kraemer HC, et al: Effect of psychosocial treatment on survival of patients with metastatic breast cancer. Lancet 2:888–891, 1989

Straus JL, von Ammon Cavanaugh S: Placebo effects: issues for clinical practice in psychiatry and medicine. Psychosomatics 37:315–326, 1996

Strauss DH, Spitzer RL, Muskin PR: Maladaptive denial of physical illness: a proposal for DSM-IV. Am J Psychiatry 147:1168–1172, 1990

Viederman M, Perry S: Use of a psychodynamic life narrative in the treatment of depression in the physically ill. Gen Hosp Psychiatry 3:177–185, 1980

Yager J, Seigfried SL, DiMatteo TL: Use of alternative remedies by psychiatric patients: illustrative vignettes and a discussion of the issues. Am J Psychiatry 156:1432–1438, 1999

Chapter 1

Integrative Psychopharmacology

A Practical Approach to Herbs and Nutrients in Psychiatry

Richard P. Brown, M.D.
Patricia L. Gerbarg, M.D.

Complementary and alternative medicine (CAM) is used by 30% of the North American population. In 1996, 60 million Americans used herbs, resulting in $3.24 billion in sales. Physicians need to understand the biochemical and evidential bases for the use of herbs and nutrients to diagnose and treat patients safely and effectively, to avoid interactions with standard medications, and to provide to patients the benefits of alternative treatments. Prior negative reactions by physicians cause many patients to conceal their use of herbs and nutrients from physicians. Patients often need reassurance that their doctor is receptive, interested, and knowledgeable about these therapies. Unless the doctor knows what the patient is taking, the patient cannot be protected from adverse interactions with other medications. Space limitations constrain us from mentioning more than a few important side effects for each compound. The *Natural Medicine Comprehensive Database*, edited by Jellin et al. (1999), presents adverse effects in greater detail.

In this chapter we indicate the quality of the evidence supporting the clinical effects of CAM. The highest level of confidence comes from well-designed, randomized, double-blind, controlled studies. The second level is based on less rigorously designed studies (on–off–on) with less elaborate design, for example, without randomization. The third level comes from open case series or clinical experience. For some compounds, there is insufficient evidence at this time to support their use; for others, evidence indicates that they are ineffective.

Credible evidence must be based on compounds produced with proper quality control and standardization—two goals that are difficult to achieve. Herbal preparations often have multiple chemical components with synergistic effects. St. John's wort, kava, and feverfew are examples of herbs having multiple active components. Consequently, it is very hard to identify which component or combination of components is therapeutic and which is ineffective or even toxic.

Because many brands are not of high quality, we provide general guidelines for choosing reliable brands. We begin with general principles relevant to CAM and follow these with discussion of clinical problem areas, including depression, bipolar disorder, anxiety, insomnia, migraine, premenstrual syndrome, menopause, hormone replacement therapy, neurologic disorders, sexual dysfunction, comorbid medical illness, side effects, and interactions.

General Issues Related to the Use of Complementary and Alternative Compounds

Many consumers pursue alternative treatments to prevent or delay health problems of aging as well as to relieve chronic health problems not adequately addressed by conventional medicine. As conventional medicines become more powerful, they often cause more serious side effects. Each year, 8,000 people in the United States die from bleeding caused by nonsteroidal anti-inflammatory drugs; others die from antibiotic allergies, acetaminophen overdoses, and adverse effects from other seemingly innocuous drugs. More and more consumers are unwilling to take such risks, at least not without trying natural medicines first. On the other hand, a current misconception that natural equals safe is belied by reports of deaths and serious illnesses caused by contaminants in unregulated herbal preparations (Ko 1998; Lightfoote et al. 1977; Schaumburg and Berger 1992) or by herb–drug interactions. To put this into perspective, in 1997 there were 8,986 suspected adverse events with herbal preparations in Europe. In the same year, the total number of adverse events from prescription medications reached 2 million (Upton 1998). In Germany, the situation is strictly regulated. The Kommission E, the German herbal equivalent of the U.S. Food and Drug Administration (FDA), reviews information about herbs and issues reports on indications, dosages, and side effects. This oversight promotes higher levels of quality in research and production while providing better information to the German public. To purchase an herb in Germany, consumers must have a prescription from a health care provider, and the German national health system pays for many herbal treatments.

Admittedly, the definition of CAM is vague. It can represent any treatment not used by the majority of allopathic physicians in the United States. This definition is arbitrary, particularly in light of the fact that many medicines were conventional treatments in other countries long before they were approved in the United States (e.g., lithium, valproate, and clomipramine).

The boundary between conventional and alternative medicine is artificial. Nearly 50% of current prescription medicines were derived from plant medicines known to European herbalists for centuries. More well-designed controlled studies are needed to transport the benefits of herbal medicine from the realm of folklore to the realm of science.

Mood Disorders

St. John's Wort

In the United States, St. John's wort (*Hypericum perforatum*) has been the most widely publicized alternative treatment for depression (Ernst 1995; Ernst and Rand 1998; Lieberman 1998a). It was popularized by the media after the publication of a 1996 meta-analysis of 23 randomized trials in 1,757 depressed outpatients (Linde et al. 1996). Thirteen studies showed that 55% of patients receiving St. John's wort improved compared with 22% receiving placebo. Three studies compared St. John's wort alone with standard tricyclic antidepressants: 64% of patients receiving St. John's wort improved compared with 59% taking tricyclics. However, the doses of tricyclics used were low (amitriptyline 30 mg/day or imipramine 75 mg/day). In two studies the improvement rate among patients receiving St. John's wort combined with valerian was higher than that of patients receiving low-dose tricyclic antidepressants (68% vs. 50%). There have been several suggestive reports that St. John's wort is helpful in the treatment of wintertime seasonal affective disorder (Hansgen et al. 1994; Kasper 1997; Martinez et al. 1994; Wheatley 1999).

Side Effects

Linde et al. (1996), in their meta-analysis, reported minimal side effects with St. John's wort. In the 13 studies comparing St. John's wort with placebo, the rate of side effects with St. John's wort was 4.8% compared with 4.1% with placebo. In other studies, 20% of patients receiving St. John's wort reported mild side effects, whereas 36% of patients receiving tricyclic antidepressants reported significant side effects. Only 15% of patients receiving St. John's wort with valerian reported side effects compared with 27% receiving placebo. Common side effects with St. John's wort are nausea, heartburn, loose bowels, jitteriness, insomnia, and fatigue. Sexual dysfunction and bruxism occur less commonly but are more frequent at high doses. Phototoxic rash occurs in fewer than 1% of people taking the usual dose (900 mg/day) but may be more likely at higher doses (Graff et al. 1997).

Preclinical studies suggest a serotonergic mechanism in the effect of St. John's wort, raising a concern that St. John's wort might interact with selective serotonin reuptake inhibitors (SSRIs) or monoamine oxidase inhibitors (MAOIs). Two possible drug interactions with serotonergic psychotropic agents were reported, but the effect of St. John's wort is so weak that other factors were far more likely to have been the cause (DeMott 1998).

Hypericin was thought to be the most important component of St. John's wort. More recent research suggests that hyperforin and napthandriones are also of significance. In one study, 147 patients with mild to moderate major depression, randomized to 6 weeks' treatment with either 5% hyperforin, 1/2% hyperforin, or placebo, had corresponding positive response rates of 70%, 55%, and 48%, respectively (Laakmann et al. 1998; Muller et al. 1998). In a subsequent study, 54 people were randomized to treatment with 5% hyperforin, 1/2% hyperforin, or placebo. The 5% hyperforin group showed the greatest changes in alpha, theta, and delta brain wave activity, a response consistent with an antidepressant effect (Schellenberg et al. 1998).

The side-effect profile of St. John's wort in higher doses is similar to that of SSRIs. Recent data suggest that at high doses St. John's wort slightly inhibits reuptake of serotonin, norepinephrine, and dopamine (Muller et al. 1997). Furthermore, there is a decrease in serotonin receptor density and a change in monocyte cytokine production of interleukin-6 (which leads to a decrease in corticotropin-releasing hormone) (Thiele et al. 1994). There is additional evidence of downregulation of β-adrenergic receptors with an increase in serotonin$_2$ (5-HT$_2$) and serotonin$_{1A}$ (5-HT$_{1A}$) subtype receptor density (Teufel-Mayer and Gleitz 1997) and in vitro binding to γ_A and γ_B receptors (Cott 1997). Other possible mechanisms involved in therapeutic effects of St. John's wort are discussed by Bennett et al. (1998).

Dosage

Studies reviewed in the 1996 meta-analysis by Linde et al. (1996) generally used 300 mg tid of 0.3% standard hypericin, although preparations differed. Since then, studies have used higher doses in the treatment of more severely depressed patients. For example, in a randomized, double-blind, multicenter trial, 209 patients received either hypericum LI 160 (Kira; Lichtwer Pharma, Berlin, Germany; a standardized research preparation) 600 mg tid or imipramine 150 mg/day for 6 weeks. Hamilton Rating Scale for Depression (Ham-D) ratings at the end of the trial were similar for both groups, although on the basis of Clinical Global Impression (CGI) ratings the group receiving St. John's wort showed 61% improvement and the group receiving imipramine showed 70% improvement. The St. John's wort group reported fewer side effects (Vorbach et al. 1997). Data suggest that higher doses of St. John's wort (more likely to cause side effects similar to those of serotonin reuptake inhibitors) are necessary in the treatment of moderate to severe depression (Wheatley 1997; Witte et al. 1995) and that the response takes longer (6–12 weeks) than with standard prescription antidepressants.

Conclusions

St. John's wort is effective in 50%–70% of outpatients with mild depression, particularly if wintertime seasonal affective disorder is present (Cott and Fugh-Berman 1998). Its side effects (i.e., insomnia, jitteriness, gastrointestinal upset, bruxism, sexual dysfunction, myoclonus), which become evident at higher doses, are similar to those of SSRIs. An ongoing study sponsored by the National Institutes of Health (NIH) and chaired by Jonathan Davidson is comparing St. John's wort with sertraline and placebo. This study should provide more definitive answers to questions about efficacy, dosing, and side effects.

We do not yet know which components of St. John's wort are the most active or how they work. St. John's wort is not reimbursed by insurance, and the price has risen with its increased popularity in the United States. However, for patients who have a philosophic preference for natural treatments or who cannot tolerate the side effects of prescription antidepressants, St. John's wort offers an effective alternative. St. John's wort is being studied for potential antiviral, anticarcinogenic, and antioxidant properties. There is considerable variability in standardization, quality, and content of brands in the United States. Most experts would recommend a brand containing 0.3%–0.5% of hyperforin and one that comes from a West German pharmaceutical firm that has done extensive research on its preparation.

The NIH-sponsored study is designed to resolve three major problems in previous research on St. John's wort: 1) the heterogeneous quality of methodology (inadequate documentation of the type and severity of the depressions studied and comparison with prescription antidepressants given in subtherapeutic doses); 2) variability in the preparations used; and 3) lack of systematic inquiry about the presence of side effects.

S-Adenosylmethionine (SAMe)

A nutrient or dietary supplement, S-adenosylmethionine (SAMe) was known only to a few physicians and researchers in the United

States until 1998. It has been used by more than 1 million people in Europe, primarily for depression and arthritis, and has been evaluated in more than 75 clinical trials involving more than 23,000 people. SAMe became available in Italy in the late 1970s, Spain in 1980, Germany in 1986, and more recently in Russia, China, and other countries, including many in Central and South America. Because of differing regulatory procedures, SAMe is a prescription medication in some countries and is sold over the counter in others. To understand the potential applications of SAMe in the treatment of diverse illnesses, knowledge of its biochemistry is essential (Baldessarini 1987).

Biochemistry

SAMe is a physiologically essential compound that some chemists believe ranks with adenosine triphosphate (ATP) as a pivotal molecule in living cells. Distributed throughout all bodily tissues and fluids, SAMe is most concentrated in the brain and liver. It is crucial to three central pathways of metabolism that stimulate more than 35 different reactions. The three major pathways are transmethylation (donation of carbon in the form of methyl groups), transsulfuration (donation of sulfur), and transaminopropylation (generation of polyamines).

Animal studies have shown that the transmethylation pathway boosts levels of neurotransmitters, including serotonin, dopamine, and norepinephrine (Otero-Losada and Rubio 1989a, 1989b). This probably contributes to the antidepressant action of SAMe (Andreoli et al. 1978; Bottiglieri et al. 1988; Curcio et al. 1978; Czyrak et al. 1992; Fava et al. 1990). Donation of carbon groups by SAMe protects dopamine neurons (Werner et al. 1999). SAMe improves nerve cell membrane uptake of phospholipids, enabling the coupling of protein receptors to second messengers within a more fluid lipid bilayer and enhancing transmission of impulses by neurons (Bottiglieri 1997). Methyl groups also help protect DNA from attack by carcinogens and reduce levels of homocysteine (Finkelstein 1998), which is a more important risk factor for heart attack and stroke than cholesterol. SAMe is vital to the production of the most important antioxidant, glutathione, as well as the secondary antioxidants cysteine and taurine (Colell et al. 1997; P. J. Evans et al. 1997).

As a precursor, SAMe donates sulfur through the transulfuration pathway, thus stimulating the proteoglycan synthesis that is necessary for cartilage regeneration in arthritis (Barcelo et al. 1987). Transulfuration and aminopropylation (i.e., donation of aminopropyl moieties) contribute to the analgesic properties and anti-inflammatory action of SAMe as well as its protection of gastrointestinal mucosa. The American diet yields insufficient quantities for both wellness and treatment supplementation. Moreover, the form of SAMe in food is not stable. Our bodies can generate only a small amount of SAMe, with the liver being the largest producer (3 g/day). Therefore, SAMe levels are most easily increased through dietary supplementation.

SAMe was discovered by Cantoni in 1952 (Cantoni 1952), but at that time no usable oral preparation (i.e., no stable salt of the molecule that would not oxidize immediately when exposed to air) was available (Stramentinoli 1987). Early studies thus employed intravenous and intramuscular formulations. The first clinical study of SAMe in the treatment of depression was done in Italy (Agnoli et al. 1976). Over the past 40 years, improvements in SAMe formulations have produced a form that is much more resistant to oxidation and to gastric enzyme degradation (enteric coated).

Lower-than-normal levels of SAMe are found in cerebrospinal fluid in some patients with depression, Alzheimer's disease Reynolds et al. 1987, 1989), Parkinson's disease treated with levodopa, disorders of folate metabolism, and other illnesses (Bottiglieri and Hyland 1994; Bottiglieri et al. 1990, 1994). Folate, B_{12}, and B_6 are necessary for efficient use of SAMe (Crellin et al. 1993). Although betaine, dimethylglycine, and trimethylglycine should theoretically raise levels of SAMe, the pathways by which these compounds exert their action are neither efficient nor clinically practical to exploit.

Evidence for Use in Depression

SAMe has been effective in numerous trials for treatment of major depressive disorder: 11 trials comparing SAMe with placebo and 14 trials comparing SAMe with tricyclic antidepressants, with more than 1,000 patients studied (Bressa 1994; Delle Chiale and

Boissard 1997; Janicak et al. 1988); and one trial using SAMe to augment response to imipramine (Berlanga et al. 1992). From 1973 to 1988, 14 double-blind European studies showed that intravenous, intramuscular, or oral preparations of SAMe were more effective than placebo and comparable with imipramine, amitriptyline, and clomipramine for treatment of major depression (Janicak et al. 1988). In 1988, the first small study by American psychopharmacologists (a double-blind, randomized 2-week trial with depressed inpatients) suggested that SAMe was effective in the treatment of depression (Bell et al. 1988).

Since 1988, double- and single-blind studies using higher doses (400 mg iv, 800 mg po, 1,600 mg po) have shown SAMe to be effective in the treatment of depression (Bressa 1994). In a double-blind trial, 30 depressed patients received 1,600 mg po of SAMe qd or imipramine (averaging 140 mg po) for 6 weeks. The SAMe group was significantly better by day 10 compared with the imipramine group. Both groups were comparably improved by week 6. One patient became mildly hypomanic for 1 week on SAMe (De Vanna and Rigamonti 1992). Other cases of hypomania were reported by Carney et al. (1988). A single-blind series of 48 patients with depression secondary to physical illness (40 of whom were medically hospitalized) compared SAMe 400 mg iv with SAMe 800 mg po for treatment of depression over a 4-week period. Both groups showed a 50% decrease in depression ratings (Criconia et al. 1994). Some patients with treatment-resistant depression may benefit from SAMe (Rosenbaum et al. 1990). In two well-designed, randomized, double-blind, placebo-controlled studies, SAMe was rapidly effective in treating postpartum depression (Cerutti et al. 1993) and postmenopausal depression (Salmaggi et al. 1993). After a week of placebo administered in a single-blind fashion, 80 women with postmenopausal depression received either SAMe 1600 mg po qd or placebo for 30 days. The SAMe group was significantly improved by day 10 (Salmaggi et al. 1993).

In a randomized, double-blind, 4-week inpatient study of SAMe, 1,600 mg/day po versus desipramine in therapeutic doses, 6 of the 11 patients taking SAMe improved compared with only 2 of the 6 patients taking desipramine. In both groups the improvement in depression correlated with SAMe blood levels (only in responders) regardless of the substance administered (Bell et al. 1994). Improvement in depression with desipramine may correlate with increases in SAMe levels, at least in the short term (4 weeks). The role of SAMe in recovery from depression and in response to antidepressants needs to be elucidated by larger and longer-term studies. Such studies could lead to a better understanding of how to use standard antidepressants with SAMe.

In 1997, at the Congress of World Biological Psychiatry, Delle Chiale and Boissard reported on two double-blind studies of SAMe. Although these were sizable studies, the post hoc analysis of SAMe effects in more severely depressed patients in both studies limits their significance. The first study compared SAMe 800 mg/day iv in 40 patients with placebo administered intravenously in 35 patients over a 3-week period. Depression ratings dropped 41% in the SAMe group and 28% in the placebo group (Delle Chiale and Boissard 1997). The second study compared SAMe 800 mg/day iv in 57 patients with clomipramine 100 mg/day iv in 65 patients for 3 weeks. Although the clomipramine group showed slightly better improvement in depression, clomipramine was far less tolerable because of its serious side effects. In contrast, SAMe was associated with a low incidence of side effects, and those that occurred were mild.

Most depressed patients receive antidepressants for long periods of time, often years. Conventional medicine has not yet tackled the issue of long-term effects of prescription drugs (Taylor and Randall 1975; Torta et al. 1988). We hope the effects are insignificant, but there are no studies, prospective or retrospective, lasting more than 2 years to assure us that these drugs are safe in the long term. Part of our confidence in using tricyclic antidepressants derives from the clinical experience of prescribing these drugs for more than 35 years. Our experience with SSRIs is less extensive (only 12 years for fluoxetine and less for other SSRIs). Considering SAMe's efficacy (comparable with that of tricyclics), rapid onset (Fava et al. 1995), low side-effect profile (does not cause weight gain or sexual dysfunction), ability to boost antioxidants, and protection of DNA through methylation, this nutrient has many advantages in the treatment of depression. Further research is needed to clarify the role of SAMe as a first-line drug in the treatment of affective disorders. In the future, perhaps SAMe will become available in large-dose preparations as a prescription drug approved by the FDA.

How to Use SAMe

Health food companies in the United States sell SAMe in 50-mg, 100-mg, and 200-mg doses. However, 200 mg is an inadequate dose to treat major depression (800–1,600 mg/day). European companies offer 200-mg, 300-mg, 400-mg, and 500-mg strengths, but these preparations are not available in the United States. In administering SAMe, keep in mind that the absorption is better on an empty stomach. Starting patients with 200 mg half an hour before breakfast and 200 mg half an hour before lunch minimizes the stimulation that some patients report in the first few weeks of treatment. This can be switched to 400 mg before breakfast after a few weeks. Patients notice an improvement in their energy level within 2 weeks. As with most medications, clinical sense indicates starting with lower doses in geriatric, medically ill, and anxious patients. If a patient has a personal or family history of bipolar disorder, lower starting doses (e.g., 100 mg once or twice a day) and careful monitoring are indicated. The dose can be raised by 200–400 mg every 3–7 days. In cases of severe depression, higher doses are required. In some studies, patients with unipolar depression have been started on SAMe at 800 or 1,600 mg/day. Problems in starting at high doses include mild, transient jitteriness, loose bowels, and headaches.

Some patients have a dramatic response to SAMe even after they have not responded to prescription antidepressants (Bell et al. 1994; Criconia et al. 1994; De Vanna and Rigamonti 1992; Kagan et al. 1990):

> Michael, a 40-year-old mental health professional, had been given trials of all available antidepressants (tricyclics, serotonin reuptake inhibitors, SSRIs, MAOIs, combinations of antidepressants and agents used to augment antidepressants) with little or no response. One week after beginning SAMe he showed significant improvement, which partially faded after 6 good months. We eventually added an SSRI to the SAMe (previous trials of SSRIs had been ineffective). With this combination the

patient recovered from his depression and has sustained remission on a reduced dose. When either SAMe or the SSRI is decreased, depressive symptoms return.

We have treated more than 30 patients with treatment-resistant depression who have responded well to augmentation of all categories of antidepressants with SAMe without adverse reactions. One randomized, double-blind study of 63 outpatients with moderate to severe major depression (Berlanga et al. 1992) confirms our clinical experience in using SAMe to augment the tricyclic antidepressant imipramine. In this study, patients were first given a 1-week placebo wash-out period, during which 23 patients improved and were therefore disqualified. The remaining 40 eligible patients were all given imipramine 150 mg/day. Half were randomized to receive either SAMe 200 mg im (equivalent to 400 mg po) or placebo im for 2 weeks. The imipramine/SAMe group showed significant improvement by day 4 as judged by decreases on depression ratings (i.e., scores on the Ham-D dropped from 25 to 17) and reduction in their use of benzodiazepines. In contrast, the imipramine/placebo group showed no significant drop in ratings by day 4. By day 10, 15 of 20 (75%) patients receiving imipramine/SAMe but only 1 of 20 (5%) receiving imipramine/placebo had scores of 13 or less on the Ham-D. By day 14, the depression ratings of both groups were comparable (Berlanga et al. 1992).

SAMe in the Treatment of Other Disorders

Fibromyalgia. Patients with fibromyalgia often see psychiatrists for treatment of pain, disability, and depression. In double-blind, controlled trials and three case series, SAMe was shown to be useful as a treatment for primary and secondary fibromyalgia in total daily doses ranging from 400–800 mg po or 200–600 mg im or iv (Di Benedetto et al. 1993; Grassetto and Varotto 1994; Ianiello et al. 1994; S. Jacobsen et al. 1991; Tavoni et al. 1987; Volkmann et al. 1997). In the most recent study, 30 patients with secondary fibromyalgia were randomized to SAMe 400 mg/day iv or placebo for 15 days. The SAMe group showed a rapid improvement in pain and depression by day 7. There were no side effects (Tavoni et al. 1998).

Attention-deficit disorder with hyperactivity. Eight adult men with attention-deficit disorder with hyperactivity (ADHD), residual type, were treated with SAMe 800 mg tid in a preliminary 4-week open trial. They were assessed with the Connors scale, a structured interview (Schedule for Affective Disorders and Schizophrenia), and other ADHD and mood scales. SAMe was beneficial in six of the eight patients. The two nonresponders had previously failed trials of methylphenidate. Side effects were minimal (mild transient headaches, loose bowels, dry mouth, stomach gas, and nausea), even on this high dose of SAMe (Shekim et al. 1990).

Parkinson's disease. SAMe may be effective in battling depression in Parkinson's disease. In one double-blind crossover study, 8 of 21 patients with Parkinson's disease showed significant improvement in depression when given SAMe (800 mg po plus 200 mg/day im). At these doses of SAMe there was no change in the symptoms of Parkinson's disease. Side effects were minimal, with mild headache, heartburn, and transient insomnia reported (Carrieri et al. 1990).

Age-associated memory impairment. SAMe may help reverse or delay age-associated memory impairment. Although Mini-Mental State Exam scores in 40 elderly patients with dementia given SAMe (800 mg/day po plus 200 mg/day im) rose from 20 to only 22 by day 60, scores on the Sandoz Clinical Assessment Geriatric Scale went from 56 to 43 (showing significant improvement in behavior, cognition, alertness, and daily activities) (Fontanari et al. 1994). The low levels of SAMe found in patients with Alzheimer's disease (Morrison et al. 1996) and other degenerative neurologic disorders in the elderly (Bottiglieri et al. 1994) warrant further study and treatment trials. Animal data suggest that by improving nerve cell membrane fluidity, β-adrenergic and acetylcholinergic receptors function like those of much younger animals (Bottiglieri et al. 1994).

Osteoarthritis. In the United States, 40 million people have radiologic evidence of osteoarthritis and are receiving medical treatment. By age 65 years, 70% of the population has documented osteoarthritis. In 20 studies of more than 22,000 people with arthritis, SAMe has been shown to exert anti-inflammatory effects equivalent to those of nonsteroidal anti-inflammatory drugs and has a 3- to 4-week period of onset. Additionally, SAMe induces proteoglycan synthesis, which results in regeneration of cartilage as documented on magnetic resonance imaging (MRI) scans in one human study and by direct measurement in rabbits in one animal study. This effect may take at least 3 months of treatment at a daily dose of 400 mg (Barcelo et al. 1987; Berger and Nowak 1987; Di Padova 1987; Konig et al. 1995).

Other disorders.   SAMe seems to reverse some of the effects of alcoholic hepatitis and cirrhosis and is used to dissolve gallstones (Frezza et al. 1990; Friedel et al. 1989; Milkiewicz et al. 1999). Preliminary studies support the use of SAMe for depression complicating alcohol and opiate withdrawal (Agricola et al. 1994). Methamphetamine depletes SAMe and dopamine levels in rat brain (Cooney et al. 1998). In several cases, we have used SAMe to successfully treat postmethamphetamine depression and drug craving.

Medication Interactions, Adverse Effects, and Warnings

After 20 years of use in other countries in more than 1 million patients, there is no evidence that SAMe interacts with other drugs, no evidence of effects on cytochrome P450 metabolism, and no evidence of displacement of other drugs from protein binding. Despite the animal data suggesting that SAMe somewhat increases levels of serotonin and dopamine, there are no clear cases of serotonin syndrome even when SAMe is combined with standard antidepressants, including SSRIs and MAOIs. Nevertheless, until adequate human studies are performed, such combinations should be monitored by a physician.

Studies comparing SAMe with placebo in the treatment of depression, arthritis, and other conditions show no more side effects with SAMe than with placebo (Berger and Nowak 1987). Side effects are generally mild and temporary, including headaches, loose bowels, anxiety, insomnia, and, rarely, upset stomach. SAMe, like tricyclic antidepressants, should be used with caution in patients with a history of cardiac arrhythmia. We have received reports of a few cases of palpitations. Drugs that affect the norepinephrine system (e.g., tricyclic antidepressants) may affect cardiac stability. When treating a patient with a serious medical problem such as cardiovascular disease, debilitation, or brittle type 1 diabetes, we recommend using lower starting doses of SAMe, smaller incremental increases on a slower schedule, and more frequent medical monitoring (Kowluru et al. 1985, 1996; Turyn et al. 1989). Standard antidepressants can exacerbate diabetes. Clinical studies using SAMe to treat depression in diabetic patients would be worthwhile. Product labeling warns against taking SAMe if there is a history of bipolar disorder.

In one study of pregnant animals, no teratogenic potential was found (Cozens et al. 1988). No evidence of mutagenic activity appeared in vitro or in vivo (animals) (Pezzoli et al. 1987). As with standard prescription antidepressants, there are no definitive prospective studies to rule out the possibility of teratogenic or neurodevelopmental effects.

The amount of SAMe passing to infants through breast milk has not yet been determined by research. However, given the high levels of SAMe normally found in infants—about three to four times higher than those in adults (Surtees and Hyland 1989)—the amount passed through breast milk may be inconsequential.

Elevation of plasma homocysteine is an independent risk factor for vascular disease. One study found low levels of SAMe in 70 patients with coronary artery disease and concluded that SAMe might be a protective factor against this disease (Loehrer et al. 1996). In a subsequent study, Loehrer and colleagues (1997) found that 400 mg/day of SAMe had a positive effect on 5-methyltetrahydrofolate, which should be useful in strategies for lowering homocysteine for prevention of coronary artery disease. Because SAMe induces the enzyme that detoxifies homocysteine, it should protect the vascular endothelium (Finkelstein et al. 1975). However, because SAMe is dependent on folate and B_{12} for its effects on lowering homocysteine, if a patient were severely folate- or B_{12}-deficient in vascular beds outside the central nervous system (CNS), homocysteine levels could, theoretically, rise and damage the endothelium. Therefore, SAMe supplementation is probably best done with adequate folate and B_{12} in the diet (R. Brown et al. 1999).

Dosage and Brands

The usual dosage of SAMe for minor depression and preventive treatment of arthritis is 400 mg/day. Doses used in the treatment of major depression range from 800 to 1,600 mg/day po. A commonly used protocol in Germany for an acutely inflamed arthritic joint is 400 mg bid for 2 weeks, followed by 400 mg/day.

SAMe preparations have been studied for bioavailability, pharmacokinetics, drug interactions, and side effects. Two forms are generally available: a butanedisulfonate form and a tosylate form. In our experience, the butanedisulfonate form seems to be superior, particularly the enteric coated form. Only two brands currently available in the United States contain the butanedisulfonate form of SAMe made by the original manufacturer in Italy. Enteric coating protects SAMe from degradation through oxidation, while stabilization is achieved by a patented process. In the United States, the stable SAMe from Italy is marketed under the brand names Nature Made (Pharmavite Corp., Mission Hills, CA) and GNC (General Nutrition Centers, Pittsburgh, PA). Analysis of several brands of SAMe with gas chromatography found that two brands claiming to have 200 mg of SAMe had none. Of five brands containing 95%–100% of 200 mg, three contained the tosylate form and two (Nature Made and GNC) contained the butanedisulfonate form with enteric coating (Faloon 1999b). If a patient has not responded to an appropriate dose of SAMe, the physician must be sure that the patient is using a potent brand.

A box of 20 tablets of 200 mg Nature Made SAMe tablets costs from $18 to $35 in drugstores, chain stores, supermarkets, and at Web sites. SAMe at a dose of 400 mg/day would cost $60 to $100 per month. Most insurance plans will not pay for an over-the-counter supplement, and, therefore, the consumer pays out of pocket.

Final Comments

Accumulated evidence indicates that SAMe in higher doses (800–1,600 mg) is perhaps as effective for major depression as tricyclic antidepressants. Studies comparing SAMe with SSRIs have not yet been performed. However, tricyclics and SSRIs have roughly equal rates of effectiveness. SAMe starts to work in approximately half the time needed for tricyclics. Studies show that SAMe has very few side effects and does not cause sexual dysfunction or weight gain. SAMe has demonstrated benefits for medical and neurologic diseases. Unfortunately, cost may be an obstacle to its use in more than a small dose for many consumers.

As a natural product, SAMe may be more acceptable to those who might not seek conventional treatment in the early stage of depression. However, patients with more significant depression may also be tempted to use SAMe to treat themselves, although the product literature warns against this. Physicians should be knowledgeable about SAMe in order to advise patients on its appropriate use as complementary treatment or as an alternative to traditional pharmacotherapy.

Nutrients

A number of nutrients, particularly vitamins, influence mood. For example, in some patients low levels of folate cause nonresponse to antidepressants (Fava et al. 1997). There are interesting differences between men's and women's responses to vitamins (Benton et al. 1995). When vitamin C, vitamin E, and seven B vitamins were given at 10 times the U.S. recommended daily allowance to a group of 129 patients for 1 year, mood improved significantly more than in a group given placebo. The same study showed that for men, higher levels of riboflavin and pyridoxine in the blood correlated with improved mood; for women, higher levels of thiamine correlated with better mood. In both men and women, improved mood was associated with levels of vitamin E and biotin (a B vitamin associated with skin and hair growth) (Benton et al. 1995).

Inositol may act as a booster of cyclic adenosine monophosphate (cAMP), a second messenger in neurons. Inositol in doses of 12–20 g/day was shown to be superior to placebo in a series of randomized trials for depression (Levine et al. 1995), panic (Benjamin et al. 1995), and obsessive-compulsive disorder (Fux et al. 1996). Inositol causes gastrointestinal side effects, including gas and loose bowels, and the dosage requirement (more than six large 650-mg pills tid) reduces compliance. One case of mania was induced at 3 g/day.

Choline has been reported to help reduce mania in a number of case reports and series. Although choline has been somewhat useful alone, a recent small case study of patients with treatment-refractory rapid-cycling bipolar disorder who were receiving lithium reported that four of six patients responded to the addition of 2,000–7,200 mg/day of free choline. The two patients who did not respond were also receiving hypermetabolic doses of thyroid medication. In one of these patients, discontinuation of thyroid medication was followed by improvement in mania. Increased intensity of the basal ganglion choline signal (measured on proton MRI) correlated with clinical stabilization. The effect of choline on depressive symptoms was variable (Stoll et al. 1996).

Anxiety

Kava

Kava, a ceremonial and social drink in the South Pacific, contains approximately 250 mg of kava lactones. Its use is constrained by elaborate rituals in Fiji, Samoa, and Tonga, where it has also been used for analgesia. Kava contains α-pyrones, a recently discovered class of potent skeletal muscle relaxants. In Germany, a dosage of 70–80 mg kava lactones tid is given for stress and muscle spasm. For milder symptoms, 60–70 mg/day kava lactones is usually sufficient. When six of the nine major α-pyrones found in kava extract are administered together in animal studies, they create a synergistic effect. Whether kava affects benzodiazepine or γ-aminobutyric acid-A ($GABA_A$) receptors is controversial. However, it has anticonvulsant properties in animal models. Kava exerts some serotonin-blocking activity and sodium channel blocking. In animal studies the primary calming effect is mediated through the amygdala. For an in-depth review of kava, see the article by Y. N. Singh and Blumenthal (1996).

Kava's traditional use as an analgesic was confirmed in mouse studies. Naloxone in doses that blocked morphine-induced analgesia did not reverse kava's antinociceptive effects. The intriguing finding that kava-induced analgesia occurs through nonopiate pathways deserves further study (Jamieson and Duffield 1990).

Efficacy

The following double-blind, placebo-controlled studies support the efficacy of kava for anxiety. In patients with generalized anxiety disorder, kava worked as well as oxazepam with no cognitive dysfunction (Lindenberg and Pitule-Schodel 1990). Improvement in "menopause-related" anxiety was observed by week 1 in 20 women receiving kava, whereas no improvement was seen in the 20 women in the placebo group during that time (Warnecke 1991). In another study, anxious patients receiving 70 mg kava lactones tid showed greater improvement compared with a placebo group by week 1 and increasingly improved over 28 days as measured by Hamilton Anxiety Rating Scale ratings (Ham-A), CGI, and self-ratings. No side effects were reported (Lehmann et al. 1996). In the longest study to date, 108 patients were randomized to treatment with 70 mg kava lactones tid or with placebo. By week 25, Ham-A scores dropped from 31 to 10 in the 59 patients who were taking kava and fell from 30 to 15 in the 49 patients in the placebo group. Significant global improvement was attained in 75% of the kava group with no evidence of dependency, compared with 50% of the placebo group (Volz and Kieser 1997). Although the patients had clinically significant anxiety, this study, like that of Lehmann et al. (1996), lacked precise diagnoses.

N. N. Singh et al. (1998) presented a randomized, double-blind, placebo-controlled 4-week study involving 60 people with subclinical anxiety of everyday life. Those given 60 mg kava lactones bid had significant improvement in interpersonal problems, personal competency, and ability to cope with environmental and cognitive stressors, whereas those in the placebo group showed no improvement.

Dosage and Side Effects

Ships' logs of vessels revisiting the Polynesian islands in the 1800s describe kava intoxication in natives and in British seamen left behind by Captain Cook. The next observed cases were reported after kava was introduced to the Maori tribe in northern Australia in 1980. Long-term kava users had poor health, with facial swelling and puffiness, scaly rash, increased patellar reflexes, and subjective complaints of dyspnea. Laboratory tests showed low levels of albumin, proteins, blood urea nitrogen, and bilirubin; increased GGTPase levels (other liver enzymes were normal); abnormal blood counts with decreased leukocyte and platelet counts; and some hematuria. Tall P waves appeared on the electrocardiograms (ECGs), consistent with possible pulmonary hypertension (Mathews et al. 1988). A case of kava toxicity was reported in the United States in 1996 when a patient tried to take himself off alprazolam (Xanax) by using kava. He became comatose while being treated in the emergency room (Almeida and Grimsley 1996). There are no studies of long-term safety, teratogenicity, or mutagenicity beyond 6 months. Kava should not be combined with alcohol or other sedatives.

Passion Flower, Chamomile, and Lemon Balm

Compared with kava, there is less scientific evidence to support the traditional use of passion flower (*Passiflora incarnata*), chamomile (*Matricaria recutita*), and lemon balm (*Melissa officinalis*) for anxiety. Passion flower contains a dihydroflavone, chrysin, that binds to benzodiazepine receptors. Apigenin, a component of chamomile, has high affinity for benzodiazepine receptors but minimal sedative, muscle relaxant, or anticonvulsant effects (D. Brown 1996). Chamomile, a member of the ragweed family, should not be used by people who have ragweed allergy. The mechanism of action of lemon balm is unknown.

Fish Extract

Extracts of *Garum amoricum* (brand names Stabilium [Life Extension Foundation, Hollywood, FL] and Adapton [Yalacta, Caen France; distributed by Smart Nutrition, Las Vegas, NV]) are used in Europe and Japan for treatment of anxiety, depression, irritability, and memory problems (Crocq et al. 1978, 1980). Hypothetically, the therapeutic effects have been attributed to neuroactive polypeptides and omega-3 fatty acids. The loading dose for *Garum* is two pills bid for 2 weeks, and then the dose is often reduced to two or three pills per day. In a double-blind crossover study, 70 college students with anxiety were randomized to either fish extract tid or placebo for 8 weeks. The group taking fish extract showed reduced anxiety by week 2; they relapsed after stopping the extract (Dorman et al. 1995).

Valerian

Valerian (*Valeriana officinalis*) is probably the best known herbal sedative. Its mechanism of action and efficacy have only weak research support. Valerian is thought to act by potently binding $GABA_A$ receptors. Four small double-blind trials for insomnia and five studies in otherwise healthy people with sleep disturbance have been reported. Valerian may require 2–4 weeks to reach its clinically significant effect. One study used valerian and hops together (hops have estrogenic effects) and compared this combination with flunitrazepam, a benzodiazepine. The authors concluded that valerian and hops did not cause deficits in attention and reaction time seen with benzodiazepines (Schultz et al. 1997). Dystonia and hepatitis from valerian have been reported, but the preparations most likely contained a mixture of ingredients, thus making it difficult to place the onus on valerian. Patient compliance is a problem because valerian tea and tablets often have a foul odor and taste.

Insomnia

Melatonin

Twenty-four patients who were already receiving fluoxetine 20 mg for major depression were randomized double-blind to either placebo or slow-release melatonin (up to 10 mg hs) for treatment of insomnia. Sleep quality and continuity improved in the group receiving melatonin. There was no difference in improvement of depression between the melatonin and placebo groups at 4 weeks. Melatonin caused no more side effects than placebo (Dolberg et al. 1998). In an open study, melatonin 3 mg po was given to 41 patients with insomnia. Sleep quality improved in 21 patients with simple insomnia and in 9 patients who had depression with melancholia. Eight of 13 patients who were also receiving benzodiazepines were able to reduce or stop their benzodiazepine use with subsequent improvement in daytime alertness. Of the 41 patients, 10 with dementia had no improvement in sleep, but 7 of the 10 were less agitated at night. No side effects occurred (Fainstein et al. 1997).

Rapid eye movement (REM) sleep behavior disorder is a chronic progressive parasomnia occurring more frequently in men and characterized by loss of paralysis during REM sleep, such that patients act out their dreams. This can result in injury to the patient or bed partner. In 50% of patients the disorder is related to neurodegenerative disorders. It is frequently found in patients with Parkinson's disease who are being treated with dopamine agonists and levodopa. In a range of neurologically vulnerable patients, stimulants, tricyclic antidepressants, and SSRIs may trigger REM sleep behavior disorder (Schenck et al. 1986). Traditional treatment by neurologists has consisted of clonazepam (0.5–2 mg hs) or carbamazepine (100 mg tid). However, these medications have drawbacks, particularly worsening cognitive function, ataxia (increased risk of falling), and other side effects. Carbamazepine can cause hepatitis, blood cell dyscrasias, and hyponatremia. In REM sleep behavior disorder, we find that 9–12 mg of melatonin is often necessary to achieve significant improvement. This application was recently supported by a case report that described the use of sleep electroencephalogram (EEG) monitoring (Kunz and Bes 1997):

> A 64-year-old man with hypertension, 7 years after having myocardial infarction, developed REM sleep behavior disorder confirmed by sleep EEG. He responded to melatonin 3 mg 30 minutes before bedtime after 5 months. Movement during sleep as recorded on sleep EEG diminished, whereas daytime alertness, cognitive function, temper, and sleep quality improved. After melatonin was stopped, symptoms gradually returned over the next 3 months.

Melatonin has been used to ameliorate insomnia in autism. Fifteen children with pervasive developmental disorders or autism with severe insomnia were given melatonin in a double-blind, placebo-controlled trial. Insomnia, irritability, alertness, and social ability improved significantly in all children taking melatonin. Three children with epilepsy gained better seizure control on doses of 2–10 mg hs (Jan et al. 1994). For a recent review of clinical studies and theoretical implications of melatonin research, see Bubenik et al. 1998.

Migraine

Feverfew

There is significant comorbidity of migraine with mood and anxiety disorders (Bott 1998). Three of four double-blind, placebo-controlled trials found that feverfew reduces the frequency and severity of migraines and associated nausea and vomiting. The negative outcome of the fourth study was attributable to its use of a preparation standardized for parthenolide (once thought to be the key sesquiterpine lactone) instead of the whole leaf extract of feverfew used by other researchers. Parthenolide is unstable and needs other components for its activity. In fact, the Canadian Regulatory Commission will only certify whole-leaf extract of feverfew as an effective medication. Spurred by uncertainty about the ideal preparation and concerned about what effects previous exposure to feverfew has on patient expectations, researchers in a recent study reduced the possibility of this bias by selecting only participants who had never taken feverfew before. In this 4-month, three-phase crossover study, 57 patients were divided into two groups. The feverfew group experienced significant reduction in migraine pain only when they were receiving feverfew.

The mechanism of activity of feverfew is uncertain. However, patients who are unable to obtain relief on standard prescription medications, many of which have undesirable side effects, may benefit from feverfew. Feverfew has virtually no side effects. Total daily doses range from 100 to 200 mg (2 to 4 pills) given in divided doses (Awang 1997; Palevitch et al. 1997).

Feverfew has additional uses, including the treatment of menstrual irregularities and arthritis. Feverfew plants from different parts of the world contain different substances. For example, the variety in Guatemala is without parthenolide and has not yet been tested in the study of migraine. This is an example of the different contexts in which experience by accomplished herbalists is needed to guide further scientific research.

Endocrine and Reproductive Systems

We discuss natural treatment for premenstrual symptoms, peri-menopausal and menopausal symptoms, and hormone replacement therapy in this section. A discussion of sexual dysfunction (with or without antidepressants) appears in the section on sexual treatments later in this chapter.

Premenstrual Symptoms

Most women who seek psychiatric treatment for perimenstrual affective symptoms do not have premenstrual dysphoric disorder but rather present with an exacerbation of an underlying mood disorder. Possible causes of affective symptoms include imbalance of estrogen and progesterone levels, which affects the functioning of several neurotransmitter systems; imbalance of calcium and vitamin D; and decrease in serotonin.

Premenstrual syndrome (PMS), including premenstrual dysphoric disorder, is a set of psychosomatic, appetitive, behavioral, and cognitive changes that occur during the late luteal phase of the menstrual cycle. Affective symptoms include nervousness, irritability, depression, crying, mood swings, and, rarely, violence. Women experience abdominal bloating and breast fullness; somatic symptoms of restlessness, headache, fatigue, abdominal pain, cramps, and back pain; and increased appetite with craving for sweets, salt, and fats (Hobbs and Amster 1996). Many women prefer to try natural treatments before taking SSRIs, which are known to be effective in the treatment of PMS. In a recent case study, Parry (1999) discussed the place of natural treatments in premenstrual disorders.

Evening Primrose Oil

Evening primrose oil (*Oenothera biennis*) is the most commonly used herbal treatment for PMS. Hypothetically, abnormal levels of omega fatty acids occur in PMS that alter sensitivity to luteal-phase prolactin and steroids. It has been theorized that the oil of

O. biennis normalizes levels of fatty acids. However, it contains predominantly omega-6 fatty acids, the amount of which is sufficient in the diet of most Americans. The American diet is deficient in omega-3, not omega-6, fatty acids. Two recent reviews of the literature concluded that studies of primrose oil have been small and poorly designed. There is no compelling evidence of improvement on evening primrose oil versus placebo (Robbers and Tyler 1999).

Magnesium

Magnesium appears to be useful in treating PMS, but only a few studies evaluating its efficacy are available. A decrease in intracellular magnesium has been found in some women with PMS. In a double-blind, placebo-controlled study, 32 women were randomized to 360 mg/day of magnesium or placebo started on day 15 of menses. The group given magnesium showed significant improvement in negative affect and arousal by the second month, followed by improvements in pain and water retention by the fourth month. There was no change in serum magnesium levels, but there was evidence of increased intracellular magnesium levels (Facchinetti et al. 1991).

B Vitamins and Minerals

B vitamins and minerals also have been reported to relieve PMS. In the most impressive study, a mixed nutritional supplement containing magnesium, B_6, vitamin E, folic acid, iron, and copper from yeast was used. In this double-blind controlled study, 40 women were randomized to the supplement or to placebo for 6 months. In the supplement group, PMS symptoms were reduced to 18% of baseline. Patients on placebo showed reduction of PMS symptoms to only 73% of baseline. There was no effect on water retention or arousal symptoms and no side effects were observed (Facchinetti et al. 1997).

B_6 is a cofactor in the metabolism of tryptophan, which is a precursor to serotonin and dopamine. It has been hypothesized that low levels of serotonin and dopamine result in high levels of prolactin and aldosterone, thus leading to fluid retention. Twelve double-blind, placebo-controlled studies of PMS treatment with

B_6 alone yielded three studies with positive results, five with ambiguous results, and four with negative results. The usefulness of vitamin B_6 treatment for PMS will remain questionable until larger and better-quality studies are done (Kleijnen et al. 1990).

Carbohydrates

Carbohydrate treatment has been used in PMS to increase the ratio of tryptophan to other amino acids. One study of a balanced carbohydrate-rich drink versus two placebos showed decreases in anger and depression 3½ hours after the drink and improved memory and decreased carbohydrate craving 1½ hours after the drink (Sayegh et al. 1995). This specially balanced, carbohydrate-rich drink is available as an over-the-counter preparation called PMS Escape (InterNutria, Lexington, MA).

Calcium

Studies exploring the effects of calcium treatment on PMS symptoms engendered the discovery of the menstrual cyclicity of calcium-regulating hormones. The results of two major double-blind controlled studies showed beneficial effects of calcium on PMS. The first crossover trial of calcium 1,000 mg versus placebo given to 33 women demonstrated significant improvement in affective, retentive, and pain symptoms in the calcium group. Appetitive symptoms improved but not significantly compared with placebo (Thys-Jacobs et al. 1989). In a second follow-up multicenter study of 466 women, calcium 1,200 mg/day or placebo was given. After 3 months, calcium reduced all PMS symptoms by 48% versus 30% with placebo. Minimal side effects included mild nausea, stomach distress, and headache. Calcium should be taken with meals to avoid stone formation (Thys-Jacobs et al. 1998).

Tryptophan

Steinberg and colleagues (1999) showed the superiority of L-tryptophan over placebo in a double-blind study. After a 2-month baseline evaluation, women with premenstrual dysphoric disorder were randomized to 3 months of either tryptophan 2,000 mg tid or placebo for the 17 days from ovulation until the third day of menses. L-tryptophan was associated with a 35% decrease in dysphoria, tension, and irritability versus a 10% decrease with placebo.

Vitex (Chasteberry)

An herb called chasteberry (*Vitex agnus castus*) has been used for nearly 70 years in Germany to treat PMS and in menopausal hormone replacement. It has been shown in vitro and in animals to bind to dopamine receptors, to inhibit prolactin release, and to increase lactation without affecting luteinizing hormone (LH) or follicle-stimulating hormone (FSH) (Klepser and Nisley 1999). In a double-blind, controlled study, 175 women were randomized to either vitex (reported to contain 3.5–4.2 mg vitex) or pyridoxine (B_6) 200 mg/day over the course of three menstrual cycles. The results of 121 of the patients who completed the study were included in the efficacy analysis; all 175 patients were included in the safety analysis. Vitex was associated with more marked alleviation of breast tenderness, edema, inner tension, constipation, and depression than was B_6. Overall, 77% of subjects receiving vitex felt that they had improved compared with 60% of those receiving B_6. Both treatments were rated as having adequate efficacy by 80% of physicians, but vitex was rated excellent by 25% of physicians versus 12.1% with pyridoxine. Of patients receiving vitex, 36% reported complete relief of PMS symptoms versus 21% of patients receiving B_6. PMS ratings decreased by 48% in both groups. Vitex side effects included headache, gastrointestinal complaints, and skin problems. No serious side effects were seen. Five women became pregnant while receiving vitex (Lauritzen et al. 1997). However, the lack of a placebo group, low statistical power, and uneven baseline prior to treatment detract from the significance of this study.

Female Menopause

Nearly 20 million women are currently experiencing menopause in the United States. This number will increase to approximately 60 million by the year 2010. Menopausal women must deal with the age-related psychologic and physical changes of menopause, which are sometimes viewed as a disease rather than a natural stage of life. Women must redefine their sexual self-image while facing increased risks of heart disease, osteoporosis, cancer, memory loss, and Alzheimer's disease. During menopause, menses become irregular and finally absent. Estrogen and progesterone decrease whereas FSH and LH levels increase. Many women endure hot flashes, vaginal dryness, mood swings, depression, insomnia, forgetfulness, poor concentration, urinary incontinence, and other symptoms (Mayo 1997).

Synthetic hormone replacement therapy (HRT) has become common practice in the United States. One component of HRT, estrogen replacement therapy (ERT), may increase the risk of breast cancer. A good deal of epidemiologic data supports a modest increase in the risk of breast cancer with long-term hormone use, particularly longer than 5 years. The 1990 Nurses Health Study followed up 121,700 women for 10 years. This study found a 40% greater risk of breast cancer in women taking HRT versus placebo. The 1995 follow-up to the Nurses Health Study found age-related increases in breast cancer risk: 40% increase in women ages 50–54 years with HRT use of more than 5 years; 70% increase in women ages 65–69 years with HRT use of more than 5 years; 32% increase in women with ERT only. A large, prospective cohort study of more than 37,105 women followed up for 11 years suggested a slightly lessened risk of breast cancer than previously thought and also indicated an association of ERT with invasive breast cancer with a favorable prognosis (Gapstur et al. 1999). Data suggest an increased ovarian cancer risk with ERT. A 7-year study of 240,073 women documented a 40% increased risk in women with ERT of 6–8 years' duration and a 70% increased risk in women with ERT greater than 11 years. Adding progesterone to ERT decreases but does not eliminate increased risk of estrogen-induced uterine cancer (Beresford et al. 1997; Colditz et al. 1990, 1995).

Common side effects of HRT include weight gain, headaches, thrombosis, fibroids, and gallstones. Positive effects include some decreased risk of cardiovascular disease, osteoporosis, and colon cancer; delay in the onset of Alzheimer's disease; and reduction of hot flashes and vaginal dryness. HRT somewhat improves visual memory and skin and muscle tone.

Many women seek natural supplements to ease the physical and psychologic changes of menopause, in part to avoid the risks associated with HRT and also to experience a more natural transition. Herbal products may be used alone or in combination for menopausal symptoms.

Soy Products

Soy products are gaining widespread use in the United States and Canada. The greater amount of soy in the Asian diet as well as cultural differences may be linked to the observation that fewer than 20% of Japanese women have hot flashes compared with 65% of Canadian women (Lock 1991). Animal studies have shown soy to have preventive effects against breast cancer and other cancers with estrogen receptors. The isoflavones are believed to have both estrogenic and antiestrogenic activity. However, no current laboratory data indicate estrogen receptor binding in vitro or enhancement of endometrial growth in ovariectomized rats (Beckham 1995; Mayo 1997; Soffa 1996). Brief reviews of soy can be found in Helmuth (1999) and Liebman (1998). We recommend use of whole natural soy products rather than isolated isoflavone preparations (such as genestein) that have different effects in young compared with older animals (Helmuth 1999).

Red Clover

Red clover (*Trifolium pratense*) is rich in isoflavones and phytoestrogens similar to those in soy products, although there are some differences. Increased levels of estrogen were measured in the blood of women who ate red clover sprouts for 2 weeks. Theoretically, red clover prevents estrogen-based cancer by blocking carcinogenic forms of estrogen at the estrogen receptor. Studies have not yet provided any laboratory data on the binding to estrogen receptors in vitro nor on uterine growth increases in ovariectomized rats (Duke 1997; Keville 1999; Soffa 1996).

Black Cohosh

Black cohosh (*Cimicifuga racemosa*) is probably the most widely used herb for menopausal symptoms. First described in the 1800s, it has been used extensively in Europe for over 60 years. By reducing LH levels, black cohosh reduces hot flashes. Most studies have not shown an estrogen-like effect. Laboratory data indicate no binding to estrogen receptors in vitro; however, it stimulates some uterine growth in ovariectomized rats. Open studies show efficacy in treating menopausal symptoms. Several controlled studies, including one double-blind, placebo-controlled study, showed efficacy equivalent to that of ERT. Unlike ERT, black cohosh had no significant side effects in the studies. Rats given 90 times the human dose for 6 months showed no toxicity. One of the major issues raised about black cohosh in the 1989 German Kommission E monographs was the lack of data beyond 6 months. Consequently, there was some concern that long-term use might increase the risk of breast cancer. However, a recent study indicated that black cohosh does not cause proliferation of breast cancer cells in culture. Furthermore, black cohosh inhibited DNA synthesis and assisted the antiproliferative activity of tamoxifen in that cell model (Fackelmann 1998; Foster 1999; Freudenstein and Bodinet 1999; Lieberman 1998b). There has been no evidence of mutagenicity or carcinogenicity.

Licorice

Licorice (*Glycyrrhiza glabra*) is an ingredient in many herbal remedies for menopausal symptoms. The active component is glycyrrhetic acid, structurally resembling adrenocortical steroids. It is reported to stimulate conversion of testosterone to estrogen and to block cancer-promoting estrogens. Used in traditional Chinese medicine, licorice is known to herbalists as the "great harmonizer." However, in excessive doses, it can rarely induce hypertension. Side effects include headache, lethargy, sodium and water retention, and potassium depletion (Robbers and Tyler 1999). Animal data suggest very strong binding to estrogen receptors in vitro. However, it does not stimulate uterine growth in ovariectomized rats. Unfortunately, there are no double-blind, controlled studies comparing its effects in the short or long term with those of HRT (Beckham 1995; Fackelmann 1998).

Dong Quai

Dong quai (*Angelica sinensis*), a traditional component in Chinese tonics since 500 B.C., has been used for menopausal symptoms and other physical problems (Mowrey 1996). It is reputed to improve blood flow, decrease blood pressure, and have antibiotic and anti-inflammatory activity. Dong quai has estrogen-like activity and can induce progesterone secretion. The water-soluble extract of dong quai regulates uterine contractions, and the essential oil relaxes uterine muscles. It has significant binding to estrogen receptors in vitro and stimulates uterine growth in ovariectomized rats (Belford-Courtney 1993; Fackelmann 1998). Chinese herbalists traditionally use dong quai in combination with other herbs. Rigorous controlled studies of dong quai alone and in combination with traditional herbs are needed.

Vitex

Vitex (chasteberry) is an herb used in combination with black cohosh, licorice, dong quai, and other herbs (see previous discussion of vitex in the treatment of PMS). Vitex increases LH production and mildly inhibits FSH, causing a shift in the ratio of progesterone to estrogen. It modulates prolactin secretion by binding to dopamine receptors. Although there are no specific studies on menopause, anecdotal reports claim that vitex alleviates affective symptoms, hot flashes, fluid retention, and weight gain. It has been used since 400 B.C. Theoretically, its ability to antagonize the effect of excess levels of circulating estrogen may protect against breast cancer. Although no side effects have been reported, vitex has very slight binding to estrogen receptors in vitro and modestly stimulates uterine growth in ovariectomized rats. It has been used to treat hyperprolactinemia, and one of the authors (R. B.) has used it to counteract prolactin elevations from antipsychotic medication (D. J. Brown 1995; Fackelmann 1998; Mayo 1997; McCaleb 1995; Soffa 1996).

Hops

In the world of natural medicine, hops (*Humulus lupulus*) are commonly used for their estrogenic effects as a component of HRT. Known to beer brewers for hundreds of years, hops are used as a sedative and are an approved sleep aid in Belgium, France, and Germany, often in combination with valerian or skull cap. Hops farmers noticed that the herb could affect those who picked it, causing fatigue and changes in women's menses. It was also known that female hops pickers had increased sex drive, whereas male hops pickers had reduced libido. Laboratory data indicate that hops bind to estrogen receptors in vitro but do not stimulate uterine growth in ovariectomized rats (Beckham 1995; Fackelmann 1998).

Blue Cohosh

American Indians used blue cohosh (*Caulophyllum thalictroides*) as a uterine tonic and to prevent miscarriages. It also has been used for menopausal symptoms. Blue cohosh has modest binding to estrogen receptors in vitro but does not stimulate uterine growth in ovariectomized rats. There are no controlled trials of blue cohosh, and its mechanism of action needs further study. (Fackelman 1998).

Questions about whether synthetic HRT or natural herbal replacement would be better in a particular case are not yet answerable based on scientific studies alone. The individual woman must gather information by asking questions, consulting medical specialists, and reading research in order to make decisions based on her best judgment, her philosophy, and her values. Some women feel more comfortable taking the known risks of synthetic estrogen and progesterone, whereas others prefer what they consider to be time-tested natural remedies, especially as recent research affirms their many benefits.

The significance of decreases in testosterone levels for menopausal women needs further research. For an in-depth discussion of the controversy over whether to treat menopausal women with testosterone, see two excellent articles in the January 1999 *Psychiatric Annals* (Bartlik et al. 1999; Rako 1999).

Male Menopause

Although prostatic enlargement is not the only symptom of middle and late life changes in men, it is the hallmark and the one for which many men take herbal supplements. Men treated for prostate enlargement often experience an improvement in sexual functioning. However, the relationship of the prostate to sexual function has not been adequately studied.

After age 45 the level of free testosterone begins to drop in men. Levels of estradiol, prolactin, and sex hormone binding globulin

(SHBG) rise. Dihydrotestosterone (DHT) rises through activity of 5-α-reductase on testosterone. Then the ratio of estrogen to testosterone rises; this occurs because the enzyme aromatase converts androstenedione to estradiol and estrone (Farnsworth 1996). The prostate is stimulated by estrogen binding to SHBG, similar to DHT. Data also suggest that estrogen inhibits the clearance of DHT. The role of the progressive drop in dehydroepiandrosterone (DHEA) sulfate after age 45 in these age-related prostate changes is not yet clear (Ding et al. 1998; Horton 1984).

The general medical treatment of benign prostatic hypertrophy (BPH) in conventional medicine involves the use of either finasteride (Proscar; Merck & Co., Whitehouse Station, NJ) or α-adrenergic blockers such as terazosin, doxazosin, or tamsulosin. Finasteride inhibits 5-α-reductase. Unfortunately, it is not as effective as the natural herbal treatments, tends to cause sexual dysfunction with 4% outright impotence, and is extremely costly ("Finasteride" 1992). The α-adrenergic blockers tend to cause tiredness, dizziness, depression, headache, abnormal ejaculation, and rhinitis ("Alpha-adrenergic blockers" 1997).

The three most studied herbal treatments for BPH are saw palmetto (*Serenoa repens*) or sabal (*Sabal serrulata*), pygeum (*Pygeum africanum*), and stinging nettle (*Urtica dioica*).

Saw Palmetto

The major components in saw palmetto are the sitosterols, which lower DHT levels and DHT binding and decrease inflammation in the prostate. Two percent of patients complain of transient effects such as headaches and stomach upset. Saw palmetto works quickly to decrease nocturia. Data from a number of studies, including one 3-year trial, suggest that saw palmetto is associated with a very significant increase in urinary flow rate and at least a 50% decrease in residual urine volume. In this study, 11% of the comparison group (patients receiving finasteride) stopped treatment because of side effects compared with only 2% of those receiving saw palmetto. Of the patients receiving saw palmetto, 80% felt very much improved in quality of life (Bach et al. 1997). The reader is referred to several reviews on saw palmetto (Carilla et al. 1984; Champault et al. 1984; Wilt et al. 1998). Other data suggest that these plant sterols may reduce cholesterol in the blood and in the liver of some patients (Laraki et al. 1993; Rau and Janezic 1992; Uchida et al. 1983). Generally, saw palmetto takes a number of months to work optimally, although many patients notice improvement within a week or two at a dose of 320 mg/day. The method of extraction of the active components may be crucial to the best results. Recent data suggest that the supercritical fluid extract is twice as effective as prior forms of the compound (Faloon 1999a).

Pygeum

Pygeum bark extract has been shown to inhibit prostate cell growth, inhibit inflammation, reduce prolactin (therefore reducing testosterone uptake in the prostate), reduce cholesterol (which reduces DHT binding), increase prostate secretions, and inhibit aromatase (which lowers estrogen/testosterone) (Barlet et al. 1990; Bassi et al. 1987; Del Valio 1974). It has no reported side effects. There is evidence of rapid improvement in nocturnal erections and sexual activity even in very elderly men (Carani et al. 1991). Pygeum doses are generally 75–150 mg/day. Perhaps the biggest issue for the long term is whether the harvesting of the bark from this very fragile tree will be sustainable (Simons et al. 1998).

Stinging Nettle

The third compound that has been extensively studied is the stinging nettle extract (*U. dioica*). Nettle extract blocks prostate cell growth receptors, blocks 5-α-reductase, inhibits aromatase, inhibits SHBG binding, and is anti-inflammatory (Lichius and Muth 1997). It has been shown to be effective alone in tests versus placebo but is better with pygeum (Krzeski et al. 1993). It is often used at a dose of 300 mg/day (Robbers and Tyler 1999).

Our own experience is that the combination of saw palmetto, pygeum, and stinging nettle produces better results than any one used alone or any two in combination. Given the greater effectiveness of the natural compounds, their negligible side effects, and their low cost compared with prescription drugs, these would seem to be reasonable alternatives for men with BPH who do not wish to take prescription medications.

Sexual Enhancement

The largest consumer groups seeking herbal or nutrient sexual enhancement are those over 40 years of age and those receiving medications that adversely affect sexual functioning. We have elected to focus on a few sexual enhancers for which there is some research evidence, frequent consumer use, or clinical experience. Because of an unfortunate gender bias, past research has been done predominantly with men. However, we have found some of the substances tested in men to be quite helpful for women.

Yohimbine

Yohimbine is both a prescription drug and a dietary supplement used to treat sexual dysfunction, particularly erectile dysfunction. Of middle-aged or older men with sexual dysfunction, 40% improved with yohimbine in double-blind, controlled conditions (Bechtel 1993; Morales et al. 1987). Some patients, particularly the elderly, cannot tolerate the side effects of anxiety, nausea, dizziness, chills, and headache. In one case series, yohimbine successfully reversed sexual dysfunction caused by fluoxetine in eight of nine men and women. Two of nine dropped out because of side effects (F. M. Jacobsen 1992). The prescription drug comes in 5.4-mg pills, and the usual dose to achieve significant improvement is 18–42 mg/day. Consumers should be aware that yohimbine content in nonprescription products is often negligible, and any improvements are most likely due to placebo effects (Betz et al. 1995). Using the prescription form of yohimbine is the surest way to obtain a quality controlled brand.

Ginseng

Asian ginseng (*Panax ginseng*) has a long history in Oriental medicine. It is often used as a sexual stimulant. There have been anecdotal reports of hypersexual behavior in patients. Animal studies have shown increases in sperm counts, testicular weight, testosterone levels, and mating counts. Studies in animal models suggest that ginseng increases nitric oxide synthesis, which is the mechanism of action of sildenafil (Viagra; Pfizer, New York, NY)

(Kang et al. 1995). One placebo-controlled study from Korea used *Panax ginseng* to treat impotence. Thirty men received *Panax ginseng* 300 mg/day for 3 months and experienced better sexual performance than 30 men receiving placebo. This study needs replication (Choi et al. 1995).

Ginkgo

Substantial literature demonstrates that ginkgo (*Ginkgo biloba*) improves blood flow to the brain, retina, leg vessels (helps relieve intermittent claudication), and penis. In one study, 50 patients were divided into two groups: 20 patients who could only achieve erections with papaverine injection and 30 patients who failed to achieve erection even with high-dose papaverine injection. All 50 men were given ginkgo for 6 months. By the end of 6 months, the first group of 20 patients was able to achieve erections without papaverine. In the second group, all 30 patients were able to achieve erections with papaverine (Sohn and Sikora 1991). The fact that this was not a double-blind, controlled study reduces the significance of this trial. Although we have used ginkgo for years to treat mild impotence in middle-aged men (after a thorough workup to rule out more treatable causes such as vascular disease, diabetes, and hormonal problems), ginkgo has not been helpful for problems with libido or orgasm. It is possible that higher doses of ginkgo might improve libido and orgasm, but the attendant increased risks would outweigh any benefits.

Arginine

Arginine supplements and sunflower seeds (which contain large amounts of arginine) have been used to treat impotence. Controlled studies using arginine to treat sexual dysfunction have not yet been performed. Nevertheless, some consumers report that arginine 9–12 g/day improves sexual function. Arginine is the precursor to nitric oxide and may alleviate angina through dilation of blood vessels to the myocardium. Some patients have taken up to 30 g/day for angina pectoris. Arginine may predispose to herpes infection in short-term use. There are no long-term toxicity studies.

Marapuama

Sexual dysfunction in men and women, whether due to aging or induced by antidepressants, can be treated with an Amazonian herb called marapuama (*Ptychopetalum guyanna*). Long used in herbal medicine as an aphrodisiac, nerve tonic, and antiarthritic preparation (Mowrey 1996), marapuama was rediscovered in modern times following a case series reported by Dr. Jacques Waynberg from the Institute of Sexology in Paris in 1990. A total of 262 men complaining of lack of sexual desire and impotence were treated with marapuama. After 2 weeks of receiving 1,500 mg/day, 62% reported enhanced libido and 51% reported better erections. There is no current research regarding the mechanism of action nor are there any controlled studies replicating this finding (Waynberg 1990). One of the authors (R. B.) has used marapuama for both men and women experiencing SSRI-induced sexual dysfunction with modest improvements in desire, arousal, and orgasmic phases.

Maca

The Peruvian herb maca (*Lepidium peruvianum* chacon), has been used for thousands of years by Andean peoples and healers. It is reported to boost energy, improve fertility, have aphrodisiac properties, improve stress tolerance and nutritional status, and relieve menopausal symptoms (Quiros and Cardenas 1997). Rat studies suggest that sterols, glucosinolates, and/or alkaloid components cause increased FSH, estrogen, and testosterone levels in female rats and increased testosterone levels in male rats (Chacon 1997; Quiros and Cardenas 1997). Recent double-blind, placebo-controlled studies suggest that maca may have positive effects on stress reduction, mood, cognition, and exercise capacity in humans. No toxicity or side effects were found in human and animal studies (J. L. Aguilar, personal communication, September 2, 1999). Use of maca may be contraindicated in patients with fibroids, estrogen receptor–related cancer risk, endometriosis, or prostate cancer. Information on maca is available from an organization called A Healthy Alternative, which can be reached by mail at P. O. Box 6013, Long Island City, NY 11106; on the Internet at www.herbalbutterfly.com; or by email at Preventmed@aol.com. Information about chemical composition and biological and clinical studies can be obtained from NaturalfaOTC@qsuiza.com.pe.

Cognitive Enhancement

Memory loss (e.g., difficulty recalling names, telephone numbers, paragraphs) begins gradually (1%–2% decrement per year) after age 20 and usually becomes significant by age 45 as measured on neuropsychologic testing (Crook et al. 1991). Drug companies call this *age-associated memory impairment* (AAMI) or *age-related cognitive decline*. Whatever euphemism is used, consumers often use the term *senior moment* for the word-finding problems and delayed retrieval experienced with age. This group of consumers in the United States and Europe is avidly interested in "smart drugs" that will improve cognitive function.

Ginkgo

Ginkgo has been used to treat Alzheimer's disease and cerebrovascular-related problems in Europe. It has been tried in a series of double-blind studies in both Europe and the United States. An excellent review of this literature has been provided by Wong et al. (1998). Ginkgo has numerous effects on the nervous system that may account for its enhancement of memory. However, memory improvements are slight at best and are dose related. A dose of 120 mg bid is necessary for observable impact in most patients with early Alzheimer's disease. Side effects are rare and can be minimized by starting at a low dose, such as 60 mg once or twice a day, and raising it gradually to the above mentioned dose. Occasionally nausea, headaches, and skin rashes occur. Because ginkgo has an effect on decreasing platelet aggregation, there has been some concern about bleeding complications. Despite the fact that millions of people currently take ginkgo in Europe and the United States, only two cases of bleeding have been reported, and neither of these is likely to be a true drug interaction because the patients were receiving far more powerful prescription medications capable of inducing bleeding.

Acetyl L-Carnitine

Acetyl L-carnitine, a neglected nutrient, is a natural compound found in small amounts in milk and meat. It is available as a prescription medication called Alcar and is used to reduce ammonia levels, which occasionally rise during valproate treatment. Studies suggest that Alcar increases energy production through the oxidative phosphorylation chain in mitochondria (Calvani et al. 1992; Di Donato et al. 1986). It has been used in studies to treat depression, particularly in geriatric patients (Bella et al. 1990), and in cognitive disorders due to cardiovascular disease (Arrigo et al. 1990). Alcar may slow the progression of early Alzheimer's disease (Brooks et al. 1998; Calvani et al. 1992). As a neuroprotector, it helps inhibit neural degeneration such as polyneuropathy (Calvani et al. 1992). Based on animal studies, Alcar may be most effective in combination with α-lipoic acid, coenzyme Q-10, and essential fatty acids to delay age-related deterioration of mitochondria (Di Donato et al. 1986; Lolic et al. 1997). However, there are as yet no studies of these effects in humans.

Selegiline

Selegiline (Eldepryl for humans [Somerset Pharmaceuticals, Tampa, FL] and Anipryl [Pfizer, New York, NY] for dogs) has been used as a treatment for Parkinson's disease. A powerful antioxidant in the brain, it has mild, amphetamine-like stimulant properties (Meeker and Reynolds 1990). Several human studies show slight improvements in cognitive function in early Alzheimer's disease (Mangoni et al. 1991). Anipryl has recently been approved for treatment of canine dementia. On the basis of one meager preliminary rat study, the alternative consumer literature often promotes selegiline as an antiaging drug. However, an antiaging effect has not been demonstrated in humans, and rat studies do not indicate what dosage might be adequate, if indeed such an effect exists.

Choline

Choline, including the form CDP-choline or phosphatidyl choline, has been used as a cognitive enhancer and as a treatment for depression. We will not discuss these applications in detail because the research is too preliminary.

Nootropic Compounds

Piracetam, aniracetam, and pramiracetam are all nootropic compounds (neural metabolic enhancers) that have been touted as "smart drugs." Although results in animal studies are intriguing, numerous attempts in human studies have not shown memory improvement. Consumers may be misled into buying these compounds, often from other countries at high prices.

α-Lipoic Acid and Coenzyme Q-10

Recent animal and human data suggest that α-lipoic acid and coenzyme Q-10 may be helpful after stroke and for ischemic heart disease (Lonnrot et al. 1998; Rosenfeld et al. 1999). The significance of these preliminary data will depend on future research (Packer and Coleman 1999).

Ginseng

Despite claims that ginseng boosts memory, four studies showed no improvement in memory or concentration with the administration of Asian ginseng (D'Angelo et al. 1986; Sorensen and Sonne 1996; Sotaniemi et al. 1995; Thommessen and Laake 1996). One 8-week study in non–insulin-dependent diabetic patients showed that ginseng 200 mg improved mood, vigor, well-being, psychomotor performance, fasting blood glucose, and glycated hemoglobin but did not improve memory compared with ginseng 100 mg and placebo (Sotaniemi et al. 1995). Another of these studies exhaustively tested memory, attention, concentration, coordination, learning, abstraction capacity, and reaction time. Danish researchers compared the effects of 400 mg/day of Asian ginseng with placebo over an 8-week period in 112 healthy middle-aged subjects. Tests were done before and after ginseng or placebo administration. The ginseng group showed improved abstract thinking and reaction times (Sorensen and Sonne 1996). One study that merits replication showed more complex cognitive enhancement with a ginkgo/ginseng combination (Wesnes et al. 1997).

Phosphatidyl Serine

Of the many nutrients studied, the most positive results have come from phosphatidyl serine (abbreviated in scientific literature to Ptd Ser or to PS in the consumer literature). Bovine-derived Ptd Ser has been studied for AAMI (Caffarra and Santamaria 1987; Cenacchi et al. 1987) as well as for Alzheimer's disease (Amaducci et al. 1988) and related conditions. More than 17 double-blind, controlled studies (many in animals) have shown clinically modest memory improvement in these conditions. For an in-depth review, see Pepeu et al. (1996). Crook demonstrated preliminary positive effects of Ptd Ser in AAMI and in early Alzheimer's disease (Crook et al. 1991, 1992). At the 1998 American Academy of Antiaging Medicine meeting, Crook presented findings on optimal dosing for rapid improvement in AAMI. A dose of 300 mg/day po for 1 month followed by 100 mg/day po thereafter led to statistically significant improvement in memory. The group that began receiving 100 mg/day required 3 months to achieve the level of memory performance of the group that was given 300 mg/day for the initial month (Donaldson 1998).

Ptd Ser, which is a small component of the inner phospholipid layer of the nerve cell membrane, may make the nerve cell membrane more fluid (as discussed previously in the section on SAMe). Bovine brain-derived Ptd Ser rich in docosahexanoic acid (DHA) (22:6n3) increased brain dopamine, norepinephrine, and epinephrine levels in animals (Salem 1989; Salem et al. 1986). In contrast, Ptd Ser from soy, which is low in DHA, did not alter catecholamine levels (Toffano et al. 1976). There are currently little data to show that soy Ptd Ser improves memory. The apparent beneficial effects of bovine Ptd Ser may be due to the cognitive enhancing effects of the omega-3 fatty acids (Hibbeln and Salem 1995). Although no cases of mad cow disease have been reported in association with bovine sources of Ptd Ser, further research is needed to determine whether this is a possibility. In the health food store, Ptd Ser is often found combined with other nutrients, such as ginkgo, despite the fact that its effect on memory is more robust than that of ginkgo. We use Ptd Ser and omega-3 fatty acids to reverse memory problems induced by antidepressants such as tricyclics, SSRIs, or bupropion with modest success.

Omega-3 Fatty Acids

Omega-3 fatty acids may prove to be the most important cognitive enhancers, particularly DHA. Low levels of DHA were associated with onset of dementia in an 8-year prospective trial of 1,200 elderly subjects. Those with low levels of DHA had a 67% greater chance of developing Alzheimer's dementia 8 years later than those with high blood levels (Kyle et al. 1998). In a recent study in Japan, Alzheimer's disease patients given DHA showed improvement in their neurologic symptoms (Nidecker 1997; Soderberg et al. 1991).

There is a flurry of recent research on the significance of omega-3 fatty acids in brain activity. Omega-3 fatty acids are critical for neural development (Crawford et al. 1993) and are important in supplementation of milk formula for babies (Jorgensen et al. 1996; Makrides et al. 1996). In formula, omega-3 fatty acids improved brain and eye development (Jensen et al. 1996) and problem solving at age 10 months (Willats et al. 1998).

Significant research shows abnormally low levels of omega-3 fatty acids in depression and aggression (Hibbeln et al. 1997; Maes 1998; Peet et al. 1998). Essential fatty acids may treat depression, although DHA has not been tested yet for this application. Hibbeln and Salem (1995) reviewed the indirect data suggesting that essential fatty acids may alleviate depression. Bovine cortex Ptd Ser improved depression in a study of 11 geriatric women. This form of Ptd Ser is nearly one-third DHA (Salem 1989). Treatment with bovine Ptd Ser 300 mg/day versus corn oil placebo significantly reduced apathy and withdrawal in 494 geriatric patients in a multicenter trial (Cenacchi et al. 1993; see also Maggioni et al. 1990).

Preliminary study suggests that omega-3 fatty acids improve the short-term course of bipolar illness and may have mood-stabilizing properties (Stoll et al. 1999). Imbalances in the distribution of omega-3 fatty acids occur in patients with schizophrenia (Saklad 1998). Also, a subset of boys with ADHD showed low omega-3 fatty acid levels (Stevens et al. 1995). These lines of research may yield new therapeutic approaches in the future. For further information, contact Martek Biosciences Corporation, 6480 Dobbin Road, Columbia, MD 21045.

The diet in civilized countries today is extremely low in omega-3 fatty acids compared with that in 1900, and Canada and the United Kingdom are moving toward requiring a minimum daily allowance of them in the diet. Omega-3 fatty acids promote cardiovascular health and reduce cardiac irritability in ischemic animal models and also improve bone density (Simopoulos 1991). A good recommendation would be to obtain approximately 25% of total calories from either omega-3 fatty acids or monounsaturated fats (as in nuts and avocados). Cold-water fish are the sources highest in omega-3 fatty acids and are the best studied. Eating fish twice a week has been shown to significantly reduce the risk of stroke. A 3-ounce serving of salmon contains 2,000 mg of DHA and eicosapentaenoic acid (EPA). Three ounces of canned white albacore tuna in water provides 1,000 mg of DHA and EPA. Rainbow trout, sardines, anchovies, caviar, mackerel, and bluefish are also high in DHA; however, smoked salmon and lox lose their omega-3 fatty acids. Patients who dislike fish may prefer fish oil capsules or liquid. α-Linolenic acid (ALA), found in plants, is partially converted in our bodies to DHA and EPA, but some people have an impaired ability to make this conversion. Flax, walnuts, canola oil, perilla oil, and dark green vegetables are all sources of ALA. Flax, the best plant source of omega-3 fatty acids, is available in flax cereals such as Health Valley's (Irwindale, CA) Golden Flax Cereal or Lifestream Natural Foods' (Blaine, WA) Flax Plus Cereal, as well as health bars such as Earthy Squares containing 20,000 mg of ALA (Earthy Foods, San Pablo, CA).

Melatonin and Dehydroepiandrosterone

Melatonin and DHEA have enjoyed a recent surge in popularity as antiaging hormones despite warnings in the medical literature. A more comprehensive, balanced view of these hormones is worthy of discussion. A great deal of scientific research has been devoted to melatonin (Bubenik et al. 1998). The best book for the lay public is *Melatonin* by Russell Reiter (1996). In animal studies melatonin delays shrinkage of the thymus with age, strengthens antibody response to vaccinations, helps immune cells fight viruses (perhaps in part by increasing natural killer cell function), and stimulates monocytes and T-helper cells.

Melatonin maintains circadian rhythms and the sleep cycle and is a powerful regulator of glands throughout the body. It has diverse clinical uses, including treatment for insomnia, phase-shift disorders, and jet lag (at least 9 mg or more are needed on the night of a flight across time zones). It is a very potent antioxidant with anticarcinogenic effects in animal and some human studies, particularly for estrogen receptor–positive tumors such as those of the breast, prostate, melanoma, and glioma. Melatonin is currently being studied as a component of oral contraceptives and for HRT. It also has been used to help ameliorate cluster headaches.

Three concerns have been raised about melatonin in the medical literature. One is that there are no long-term data for its use in insomnia. Ironically, some articles that raise this issue do not address the fact that there are also no data on the long-term use of conventional sedative-hypnotics and that some data suggest that those prescription medications cause long-term toxicity to the brain in animals and humans (Golombok et al. 1998). Considering its well-demonstrated antioxidant properties, melatonin has more benefits than any currently available prescription hypnotic. The second issue is whether commercial preparations are pharmaceutically pure. *The Medical Letter* ("Melatonin" 1995) reported that four of six samples of melatonin off the shelf had impurities that were hard to define. This means that consumers need to choose supplements that are from mainstream companies and that indicate that they contain pharmaceutical-grade melatonin. Unfortunately, there are only meager data to guide dosing. The doses for insomnia range from 0.3 to 12 mg or more. The third issue is whether giving high doses of melatonin leads to abnormally high supraphysiologic levels of melatonin. This may be of less concern in light of recent data suggesting that the overuse of nighttime lighting in our society leaves us with decreased levels of melatonin, thus contributing to an increased cancer risk (Raloff 1998).

DHEA has been featured as a fountain of youth by some media writers. In primates, the adrenal glands are the primary producers of DHEA sulfate. The ovaries also contribute some production. In humans, DHEA levels rise at puberty, leading to a high level in adulthood that then drops steadily after age 40. For years it was thought to be merely a precursor for androgens and estrogens in the periphery of the body, a so-called buffer hormone. It has significant neurologic effects with evidence in humans and animals of improved memory and brain activation on EEG. In a case report, DHEA was used to treat depression (Bonnet and Brown 1990). Wolkowitz and colleagues (1999) reported that 22 patients with a partially resistant major depression were treated with DHEA, up to 90 mg/day for 6 weeks alone or in addition to antidepressants. Five of 11 patients receiving DHEA responded versus none of the 11 patients receiving placebo. In a double-blind, randomized crossover study, 17 men and women ages 45–63 years with midlife dysthymia were treated with 3 weeks of DHEA 90 mg/day, 3 weeks of DHEA 450 mg/day, and 6 weeks of placebo. Fifteen patients who completed the study showed a robust improvement in mood with DHEA compared with those receiving placebo. After only 3 weeks of treatment with 90 mg/day DHEA, 60% responded to DHEA compared with 20% to placebo (Bloch et al. 1999). Internists who have used this "alternative" treatment for years have generally increased DHEA and DHEA sulfate levels to the high end of normal range for patients ages 20–30 years (Wolkowitz et al. 1999). Our clinical experience is that patients with low DHEA levels for age, such as menopausal women (particularly those who have had ovaries or adrenal glands removed) and geriatric patients with debilitating medical or neurologic disease, are likely to respond with improvements in mood and memory.

In animal models, DHEA has been shown to improve insulin sensitivity, lupus erythematosus, rheumatoid arthritis, and the speed of burn healing. DHEA improves bone density in menopausal women and in aged rats. In healthy elderly patients, long-term studies showed improvements in strength, sleep, coping, joint mobility, lean body mass, and improved libido in men. However, not all studies agree, and further research is needed (Skolnick 1996).

DHEA is probably best used under medical supervision with the goal of restoring low levels to a physiologic level. A concern has been that DHEA might cause increased levels of DHT, although recent data suggest otherwise. Many alternative medicine practitioners recommend antioxidants that help improve the prostate, such as soy, lycopene, and the 5-α-reductase inhibitor saw palmetto. Serial prostate-specific antigen levels may be checked. Some data suggest that DHEA slightly increases estrogen levels in women. If patients choose to take this hormone, they should obtain pharmaceutical-grade DHEA.

Obesity

Weight gain can be triggered or aggravated by psychotropic medication. Weight loss agents are important, particularly for overall health and patient compliance. Of the many products in health food stores, only two have documented and observable effects in clinical practice: chromium picolinate and the combination of ephedrine and caffeine.

Chromium Picolinate

The mineral chromium in picolinate form enables insulin to pass through capillary walls more easily and reduces insulin resistance. It also helps cells use glucose more efficiently, prevents formation of abnormal lipids, and raises DHEA levels. The preponderance of studies show that chromium reduces body fat even without exercise. Chromium picolinate combined with a weight training program produces an even greater reduction in body fat and some increase in muscle mass, mainly in women. Chromium reverses some markers of atherosclerosis, including lowering total and low- and high-density lipoprotein cholesterol in human and animal studies. In animal and human studies, chromium has been used to reverse diabetes, including that of pregnancy. Two replicated studies showed that chromium picolinate leads to a 25% longer life span and 25% less body fat in rats compared with placebo or another form of chromium. Data also suggest that in menopausal women, chromium picolinate raises DHEA and estrogen levels, improves bone density, and reverses urinary calcium loss. For a fuller review of these studies, including the controversy over toxicity, see *Chromium Picolinate: Everything You Need to Know* by G. Evans (1996). Studies reporting weight loss have used 400–600 µg/day. A study of adult-onset type 2 diabetic patients showed that 500 µg bid was effective (Anderson et al.

1997). We have used chromium picolinate to reverse weight gain from antidepressants in clinical practice and have noted that it often improves mood. This was supported by a recent small case series of single-blind, on–off–on, open-label trials. Five patients with dysthymia in partial remission, four of whom were receiving sertraline and one of whom was receiving nortriptyline, achieved full remission when given chromium picolinate 400 µg/day (McLeod et al. 1999).

Ephedrine–Caffeine Combination

Confirming earlier primate studies (Ramsey et al. 1998), four major double-blind, placebo-controlled studies showed the combination of ephedrine and caffeine to be superior to either placebo or dexfenfluramine for weight loss in humans (Astrup et al. 1992; Breum et al. 1994; Daly et al. 1993; Toubro et al. 1993). Ephedrine with caffeine induces appetite suppression within 3 weeks. Its long-term effect is to reduce body fat, seemingly by increasing fat burning and heat production. This begins by week 3 and increases with time. In these studies, patients tolerated the stimulant effect extremely well if they received low doses of the combination initially and doses were increased gradually. However, many precautions must be followed in considering ephedrine and caffeine. Contraindications include cardiovascular disease, the use of asthma medications, psychosis, prostate disease, and others.

Herb–Drug Interactions

Our discussion of significant interactions between drugs and herbs must be brief and selective. John Neeld Jr., president of the American Society of Anesthesiologists, recently warned that a number of anesthesiologists have anecdotally reported significant changes in heart rate and blood pressure, particularly in patients taking St. John's wort, ginkgo, and ginseng. He recommended stopping herbal medications 2–3 weeks before surgery (Voelker 1999). Herbs that can affect bleeding time (e.g., feverfew, garlic, ginkgo, ginger, and ginseng) should not be used with warfarin, and use should be stopped prior to surgery. The use of St. John's wort with medications that have significant action on the serotonergic system (SSRIs or MAOIs) should be avoided at present because of limited testing. Valerian and kava should not be used with other sedating medications because of the potential for additive sedative effects. Evening primrose oil and borage oil (a source of omega-3 fatty acids) should not be used with anticonvulsants because they may lower seizure thresholds. Patients should be warned to avoid immunostimulants such as echinacea and astragalus when taking immunosuppressants such as steroids and cyclosporine for transplantation. Licorice may counteract the therapeutic effects of spironolactone. Chromium picolinate, ginseng, bitter melon, and fenugreek may affect blood glucose levels. Herbal laxatives or licorice, by depleting potassium, may affect the therapeutic action of digoxin, β-blockers, and diuretics. For a more extensive review see Miller (1998).

Athletic Enhancement

Another area that we cannot cover in this chapter is the use of athletic enhancers. Many patients, particularly adolescents, may try substances such as androstenedione despite the absence of adequate scientific information documenting safety in this age population. Physicians will find information on this subject in *The Medical Letter* ("Creatinine and androstenedione" 1998).

Physician Education

Patients need help understanding how to find quality alternative therapy products whose efficacy has adequate clinical and research support. Yager et al. (1999) present useful guidelines for discussing alternative treatments with patients. Physicians can begin to educate themselves with a recent review article on the most common herbal remedies used in North American populations (Wong et al. 1998). The Herb Research Foundation, started by Andrew Weil in coordination with the American Botanical Council, publishes *Herbalgram*, which features reviews and abstracts of recent studies in scientific journals as well as area reviews. Monographs on any herb may be obtained from the Herb Research Foundation (phone number 303-449-2265) with a small fee for members. For physicians, *The Green Pharmacy* by James Duke (1997) and *Tyler's Herbs of Choice* by James Robbers and Varro Tyler (1999) are extremely helpful. The new *Natural Medicines Comprehensive Database* (Jellin et al. 1999) is the book to read when faced with a patient taking an esoteric herb. Clinicians may contact The Natural Product Research Consultants at 973-762-0840 or The American Botanical Council at 512-926-4900. The NIH is building a dietary supplement database accessible on the Internet at www.nalusda.gob/fmic-IBIDS.

We encourage psychiatrists to become knowledgeable about CAM—once an ancient form of healing, now a rapidly growing branch of modern medicine.

References

Agnoli A, Andreoli V, Casacchia M, et al: Effect of *S*-adenosyl-L-methionine (SAMe) upon depressive symptoms. J Psychiatr Res 13:43–54, 1976

Agricola R, Dalla Verde G, Urani R, et al: *S*-adenosyl-L-methionine in the treatment of major depression complicating chronic alcoholism. Current Therapeutic Research, Clinical and Experimental 55:83–92, 1994

Almeida JC, Grimsley EW: Coma from the health food store: interaction between kava and alprazolam. Ann Intern Med 125:940–941, 1996

Alpha-adrenergic blockers. The Medical Letter 39:96, 1997

Amaducci L and the SMID Group: Phosphatidylserine in the treatment of Alzheimer's disease: results of a multicenter study. Psychopharmacol Bull 24:130–134, 1988

Anderson RA, Cheng N, Bryden NA, et al: Elevated intakes of supplemental chromium improve glucose and insulin variables in individuals with type 2 diabetes. Diabetes 46:1786–1791, 1997

Andreoli VM, Maffei F, Tonon GC: *S*-Adenosyl-L-methionine (SAMe) blood levels in schizophrenia and depression [in Italian], in Transmethylation and the Central Nervous System. New York, Springer-Verlag, 1978, pp 147–150

Arrigo A, Casale R, Buonocore M, et al: Effects of acetyl-L-carnitine on reaction times in patients with cerebrovascular insufficiency. Int J Clin Pharmacol Res 10:133–137, 1990

Astrup A, Breum L, Toubro S, et al: The effect and safety of an ephedrine/caffeine compound compared to ephedrine, caffeine, and placebo in obese subjects on an energy restricted diet: a double-blind trial. Int J Obes Relat Metab Disord 16:269–277, 1992

Awang DVC: Feverfew trials: the promise of—and the problem with—standardized botanical extracts. Herbalgram 41:16–17, 1997

Bach D, Schmitt M, Ebeling L: Phytopharmaceutical and synthetic agents in the treatment of benign prostatic hyperplasia (BPH). Phytomedicine 4:309–313, 1997

Baldessarini RJ: Neuropharmacology of S-adenosyl-L-methionine. Am J Med 83(5A):95–103, 1987

Barcelo HA, Wiemeyer JC, Sagasta CL, et al: Effect of S-adenosylmethionine on experimental osteoarthritis in rabbits. Am J Med 83(5A):55–59, 1987

Barlet A, Albrecht J, Aubert A, et al: Efficacy of *Pygeum africanum* extract in the treatment of micturitional disorders due to benign prostatic hyperplasia: evaluation of objective and subjective parameters. A multicenter, randomized, double-blind trial. Wien Klin Wochenschr 102(22):667–673, 1990

Bartlik B, Legere R, Andersson L: The combined use of sex therapy and testosterone replacement therapy for women. Psychiatric Annals 29:27–33, 1999

Bassi P, Artibani W, De Luca V, et al: Standardized *Pygeum africanum* extract in the treatment of benign prostatic hypertrophy: a controlled clinical study versus placebo. Minerva Urol Nefrol 39:45–50, 1987

Bechtel S: The Practical Encyclopedia of Sex and Health. Emmaus, PA, Rodale Press, 1993, pp 343–346

Beckham N: Phyto-oestrogens and compounds that affect oestrogen metabolism, part II. Aust J Med Herb 7(2):27–33, 1995

Belford-Courtney R: Comparison of Chinese and Western users of Angelica sinesis. Aust J Med Herb 5(4):87–91, 1993

Bell KM, Plon L, Bunney WE Jr, et al: S-Adenosylmethionine treatment of depression: a controlled clinical trial. Am J Psychiatry 145:1110–1114, 1988

Bell KM, Potkin SG, Carreon D, et al: S-Adenosylmethionine plasma levels in major depression: changes with drug treatment. Acta Neurol Scand 154:15–18, 1994

Bella R, Biondi R, Raffaele R, et al: Effect of acetyl L-carnitine on geriatric patients suffering from dysthymic disorders. Int J Clin Pharmacol Res 10:355–360, 1990

Benjamin J, Levine J, Fux M, et al: Double-blind, placebo-controlled, crossover trial of inositol treatment for panic disorder. Am J Psychiatry 152:1084–1086, 1995

Bennett DA Jr, Phun L, Polk JF, et al: Neuropharmacology of St John's wort (*Hypericum*). Ann Pharmacother 32:1201–1208, 1998

Benton D, Haller J, Fordy J: Vitamin supplementation for 1 year improves mood. Neuropsychobiology 32:98–105, 1995

Beresford SA, Weiss NS, Voigt LF, et al: Risk of endometrial cancer in relation to use of oestrogen combined with cyclic progestagen therapy in postmenopausal women. Lancet 349:458–461, 1997

Berger R, Nowak H: A new medical approach to the treatment of osteoarthritis: report of an open phase IV study with ademetionine (*Gumbaral*). Am J Med 83(5A):84–88, 1987

Berlanga C, Ortega-Soto HA, Ontiveros M, et al: Efficacy of S-adenosyl-L-methionine in speeding the onset of action of imipramine. J Psychiatr Res 44:257–262, 1992

Betz S, White KD, Der Marderosian AH: Gas chromatographic determination of yohimbine in commercial yohimbe products. J AOAC Int 78:1189–1194, 1995

Bloch M, Schmidt PJ, Danaceau MA, et al: Dehydroepiandrosterone treatment of midlife dysthymia. Biol Psychiatry 45:1533–1541, 1999

Bonnet KA, Brown RP: Cognitive effects of DHEA replacement therapy, in The Biological Role of Dehydroepiandrosterone. Edited by Kalimi MY, Regelson W. New York, Walter de Gruyter, 1990, pp 65–79

Bott AD: The comorbidity of mood and anxiety disorders: implications for treatment. Primary Psychiatry 5(11):77–86, 1998

Bottiglieri T: Ademetionine (S-adenosylmethionine) neuropharmacology: implications for drug therapies in psychiatric and neurological disorders. Expert Opinion in Investigational Drugs 6:417–426, 1997

Bottiglieri T, Hyland K: S-Adenosylmethionine levels in psychiatric and neurological disorders: a review. Acta Neurol Scand Suppl 154:19–26, 1994

Bottiglieri T, Chary TKN, Laundy M, et al: Transmethylation and depression. Ala J Med Sci 25:296–300, 1988

Bottiglieri T, Godfrey P, Flynn T, et al: Cerebrospinal fluid S-adenosylmethionine in depression and dementia: effects of treatment with parenteral and oral S-adenosylmethionine. J Neurol Neurosurg Psychiatry 53:1096–1098, 1990

Bottiglieri T, Hyland K, Reynolds EH: The clinical potential of ademetionine (S-adenosylmethionine) in neurological disorders. Drugs 48:137–152, 1994

Bressa GM: S-Adenosyl-L-methionine (SAMe) as antidepressant: meta-analysis of clinical studies. Acta Neurol Scand Suppl 154:7–14, 1994

Breum L, Pedersen JK, Ahlstrom F, et al: Comparison of an ephedrine/caffeine combination and dexfenfluramine in the treatment of obesity: a double-blind multi-center trial in general practice. Int J Obes Relat Metab Disord 18:99–103, 1994

Brooks JO, Yesavage JA, Carta A, et al: Acetyl-L-carnitine slows decline in younger patients with Alzheimer's disease: a reanalysis of a double-blind, placebo-controlled study using the trilinear approach. Int Psychogeriatr 10:193–203, 1998

Brown D: Anti-anxiety effects of chamomile compounds. Herbalgram 39:19, 1996

Brown DJ: *Vitex agnus castus*: clinical monograph. Townsend Letter for Doctors and Patients, 1995, pp 138–142

Brown R, Bottiglieri T, Colman C: Stop Depression Now. New York, Penguin/Putnam, 1999

Bubenik GA, Blask DE, Brown GM, et al: Prospects of the clinical utilization of melatonin. Biol Signals Recept 7:195–219, 1998

Caffarra P, Santamaria V: The effects of phosphatidylserine in patients with mild cognitive decline: an open trial. Clinical Trials Journal 24:109–114, 1987

Calvani M, Carta A, Caruso G, et al: Action of acetyl L-carnitine in neurodegeneration and Alzheimer's disease. Ann N Y Acad Sci 663:483–486, 1992

Cantoni GL: The nature of the active methyl donor formed enzymatically from L-methionine and adenosinetriphosphate. Journal of the American Chemical Society 74:2942–2943, 1952

Carani C, Salvioli V, Scuteria A, et al: Urological and sexual evaluation of treatment of benign prostatic disease using *Pygeum africanum* at high doses. Archivio Italiano di Urologia, Nefrologia, Andrologia 63:341–345, 1991

Carilla D, Briley M, Faurin F, et al: Binding of permixon, a new treatment for prostatic benign hyperplasia to the cytosolic androgen receptor in the rat prostate. J Steroid Biochem 20:251–253, 1984

Carney MWP, Chary TKN, Bottiglieri T, et al: Switch and S-adenosylmethionine. Ala J Med Sci 25:316–319, 1988

Carrieri PB, Indaco A, Gentile S, et al: S-Adenosylmethionine treatment of depression in patients with Parkinson's disease: a double-blind crossover study versus placebo. Current Therapeutic Research, Clinical and Experimental 48:154–160, 1990

Cenacchi T, Baggio C, Palin E: Human tolerability of oral phosphatidylserine assessed through laboratory examinations. Clinical Trials Journal 24:125–130, 1987

Cenacchi T, Bertoldin T, Faarina C, et al: Cognitive decline in the elderly: a double-blind, placebo controlled multicenter study of the efficacy of phosphatidylserine administration. Aging (Milano) 5:123–133, 1993

Cerutti R, Sichel MP, Perin M, et al: Psychological distress during puerperium: a novel therapeutic approach using S-adenosylmethionine. Current Therapeutic Research, Clinical and Experimental 53:707–716, 1993

Chacon GA: La importancia de *Lepidium peruvianum Chacon* ("Maca") en la alimentacion y salud humano y animal 2,000 anos antes y despues de cristo y en el siglo XXI. Unpublished dissertation, Universidad Nacional Mayor de San Marcos, Lima, Peru, 1997

Champault G, Patel JC, Bonnard AM: A double bind trial of an extract of the plant *Seronoa repens* in benign prostatic hyperplasia. Br J Clin Pharmacol 18:461–462, 1984

Choi HK, Seong DH, Rha KH: Clinical efficacy of Korean red ginseng for erectile dysfuntion. Int J Impot Res 7(3):181–186, 1995

Colditz GA, Stampfer MJ, Willet WC, et al: Prospective study of estrogen replacement therapy and risk of breast cancer in postmenopausal women. JAMA 264:2648–2653, 1990

Colditz GA, Hankinson SE, Hunter DJ, et al: The use of estrogens and progestins and the risk of breast cancer in postmenopausal women. N Engl J Med 332:1589–1593, 1995

Colell A, Garcia-Ruiz C, Morales A, et al: Transport of reduced glutathione in hepatic mitochondria and mitoplasts from ethanol-treated rats: effect of membrane physical properties and S-adenosyl-L-methionine. Hepatology 26:699–708, 1997

Cooney CA, Wise CK, Poirier LA, et al: Methamphetamine treatment affects blood and liver S-adenosylmethionine (SAM) in mice: correlation with dopamine depletion in the striatum. Ann N Y Acad Sci 844:191–200, 1998

Cott JM: In vitro receptor binding and enzyme inhibition by *Hypericum perforatum* extract. Pharmacopsychiatry 30 (suppl 2):108–112, 1997

Cott JM, Fugh-Berman A: Is St John's wort (*Hypericum perforatum*) an effective antidepressant? J Nerv Ment Dis 186:500–501, 1998

Cozens DD, Barton SJ, Clark R, et al: Reproductive toxicity studies of Ademetionine. Arzneimittelforschung 38:1625–1629, 1988

Crawford MA, Doyle W, Leaf A, et al: Nutrition and neurodevelopmental disorders. Nutrition and Health 9:81–97, 1993

Creatinine and androstenedione—two "dietary supplements." The Medical Letter 40:105–106, 1998

Crellin R, Bottiglieri T, Reynolds EH: Folates and psychiatric disorders. Drugs 45:623–636, 1993

Criconia AM, Araquistain JM, Daffina N, et al: Results of treatment with S-adenosyl-L-methionine in patients with major depression and internal illnesses. Current Therapeutic Research, Clinical and Experimental 55:666–674, 1994

Crocq L, Bugard P, Viaud P: Fatigue Study Group inquiry into asthenia in general practice. Psychologie Medicale 10:1943–1953, 1978

Crocq L, Bugard P, Viaud P: Treatment of astheno-depressive conditions by Minaprine: multi-center study of 248 cases assessed by Fatigue Study Group Scale #4. Psychologie Medicale 12:643–661, 1980

Crook TH, Tinkelberg J, Petrie W, et al: Effects of phosphatidylserine in age-associated memory impairment. Neurology 41:644–649, 1991

Crook TH, Petrie W, Wells C, et al: Effects of phosphatidylserine in Alzheimer's disease. Psychopharmacol Bull 28:61–66, 1992

Curcio M, Catto E, Stramentinoli G, et al: Effect of S-adenosyl-L-methionine on serotonin metabolism in rat brain. Progress in Neuropsychopharmacology 2(2):65–71, 1978

Czyrak A, Rogoz Z, Skuza G, et al: Antidepressant activity of S-adenosyl-L-methionine in mice and rats. J Basic Clin Physiol Pharmacol 3:1–17, 1992

Daly PA, Krieger DR, Dulloo AG, et al: Ephedrine, caffeine and aspirin: safety and efficacy for treatment of human obesity. Int J Obes Relat Metab Disord 17 (suppl 1):73–78, 1993

D'Angelo L, Grimaldi R, Caravaggi M, et al: A double blind, placebo controlled study on the effect of standardized ginseng extract on psychomotor performance in healthy volunteers. J Ethnopharmacol 16:15–22, 1986

De Vanna M, Rigamonti R: Oral S-adenosyl-L-methionine in depression. Current Therapeutic Research, Clinical and Experimental 52:478–485, 1992

Del Valio B: The use of a new drug in the treatment of chronic prostatitis. Minerva Urologica 26:87–94, 1974

Delle Chiale R, Boissard G: Paper presented at the World Biological Psychiatry Congress, Abstract 90-56. Biol Psychiatry 42(suppl 1):245S, 1997

DeMott K: St. John's wort tied to serotonin syndrome. Clinical Psychiatry News, March 1998, p 28

Di Benedetto P, Iona LG, Zidarich V: Clinical evaluation of *S*-adenosyl-L-methionine versus transcutaneous electrical nerve stimulation in primary fibromyalgia. Current Therapeutic Research, Clinical and Experimental 53:222–229, 1993

Di Donato S, Frerman FE, Rimoldi MS, et al: Systemic carnitine deficiency due to lack of electron transfer flavoprotein: ubiquinone oxidoreductase. Neurology 36:957–963, 1986

Di Padova C: *S*-Adenosylmethionine in the treatment of osteoarthritis: review of the clinical studies. Am J Med 83(5A):60–65, 1987

Ding VD, Moller DE, Feeney WP, et al: Sex hormone–binding globulin mediates prostate androgen receptor action via a novel signaling pathway. Endocrinology 139:213–218, 1998

Dolberg OT, Hirschmann S, Grunhaus L: Melatonin for the treatment of sleep disturbances in major depressive disorder. Am J Psychiatry 155:1119–1121, 1998

Donaldson T: Exploring the future. Life Extension Journal, April 1998, pp 37–38

Dorman T, Bernard L, Glaze P, et al: The effectiveness of *Garum amoricum* (stabilium) on reducing anxiety in college students. Journal of Advances in Medicine 8:193–200, 1995

Duke JA: The Green Pharmacy. Emmaus, PA, Rodale Press, 1997

Ernst E: St. John's wort, an antidepressant? A systematic criteria-based review. Phytomedicine 2:67–71, 1995

Ernst E, Rand JI, Stevinson C: Complementary therapies for depression: an overview. Arch Gen Psychiatry 55:1026–1032, 1998

Evans G: Chromium Picolinate: Everything You Need to Know. Garden City Park, NY, Avery Publishing Group, 1996

Evans PJ, Whiteman M, Tredger JM, et al: Antioxidant properties of *S*-adenosyl-L-methionine: a proposed addition to organ storage fluids. Free Radic Biol Med 23:1002–1008, 1997

Facchinetti F, Borella P, Sances G, et al: Oral magnesium successfully relieves premenstrual mood changes. Obstet Gynecol 78:177–181, 1991

Facchinetti F, Nappi RE, Sances MG, et al: Effects of a yeast-based dietary supplementation on premenstrual syndrome. Gynecol Obstet Invest 43:120–124, 1997

Fackelman K: Medicine for menopause. Science News 153:392–393, 1998

Fainstein I, Bonetto AJ, Brusco LI, et al: Effects of melatonin in elderly patients with sleep disturbance: a pilot study. Current Therapeutic Research, Clinical and Experimental 58:990–1000, 1997

Faloon M: BPH: the other side of the coin. Life Extension Journal, February 1999a, pp 12–17

Faloon M: Counterfeit supplements. Life Extension Journal, September 1999b, pp 7–9

Farnsworth WE: Roles of estrogen and SHBG in prostate physiology. Prostate 28(1):17–23, 1996

Fava M, Rosenbaum JF, MacLaughlin R, et al: Neuroendocrine effects of S-adenosyl-L-methionine, a novel putative antidepressant. J Psychiatr Res 24:177–184, 1990

Fava M, Giannelli A, Rapisarda V, et al: Rapidity of onset of the antidepressant effect of parenteral S-adenosyl-L-methionine. Psychiatry Res 56:295–297, 1995

Fava M, Borus JS, Alpert JE, et al: Folate, vitamin B_{12}, and homocysteine in major depressive disorder. Am J Psychiatry 154:426–428, 1997

Finasteride. The Medical Letter 34:83, 1992

Finkelstein JD: The metabolism of homocysteine: pathways and regulation. Eur J Pediatr 157(suppl):S40–S44, 1998

Finkelstein JD, Kyle WE, Martin JJ, et al: Activation of cystathionine synthase by adenosylmethionine and adenosylethionine. Biochem Biophys Res Commun 66:81–87, 1975

Fontanari D, Di Palma C, Giorgetti G, et al: Effects of S-adenosyl-L-methionine on cognitive and vigilance functions in the elderly. Current Therapeutic Research, Clinical and Experimental 55:682–689, 1994

Foster S: Black cohosh Cimicifugae racemosa: a literature review. Herbalgram 45:36–49, 1999

Freudenstein J, Bodinet C: Influence of an isopropanolic aqueous extract of Cimicifugae racemosa rhizoma on the proliferation of MCF-7 cells. Presentation at the 23rd International LOF-Symposium on Phytoestrogens, University of Ghent, Belgium, January 15, 1999

Frezza M, Surrenti C, Manzillo G, et al: Oral S-adenosyl-methionine in the symptomatic treatment of intrahepatic cholestasis: a double-blind, placebo-controlled study. Gastroenterology 99:211–215, 1990

Friedel HA, Goa KL, Benfield P: S-Adenosyl-methionine: a review of its pharmacological properties and therapeutic potential in liver dysfunction and affective disorders in relation to its physiological role in cell metabolism. Drugs 38:389–416, 1989

Fux M, Levine J, Aviv A, et al: Inositol treatment of obsessive-compulsive disorder. Am J Psychiatry 153:1219–1221, 1996

Gapstur SM, Morrow M, Sellers TA: Hormone replacement therapy and risk of breast cancer with a favorable histology: results of the Iowa Women's Health Study. JAMA 281:2091–2097, 1999

Golombok S, Moodley P, Lader M: Cognitive impairment in long-term benzodiazepine users. Psychol Med 18:365–374, 1998

Graff A, Williamson E: St. John's wort, *Hypericum perforatum*, in American Herbal Pharmacopoeia and Therapeutic Compendium. Edited by Upton R. Santa Cruz, CA, American Herbal Pharmacopoeia, 1997

Grassetto M, Varotto A: Primary fibromyalgia is responsive to *S*-adenosyl-L-methionine. Current Therapeutic Research, Clinical and Experimental 55:797–806, 1994

Gruenwald J, Brendler BA, Jaenicke C, et al (eds): PDR for Herbal Medicines. Montvale, NJ, Medical Economics Data, 1998

Hansgen KD, Vesper J, Ploch M: Multicenter double-blind study examining the antidepressant effectiveness of the hypericum extract L160. J Geriatr Psychiatry Neurol 7(suppl 1):S15–S18, 1994

Helmuth L: Nutritionists debate soy's health benefits. Science News 155:262, 1999

Hibbeln JR, Salem N Jr: Dietary polyunsaturated fatty acids and depression: when cholesterol does not satisfy. Am J Clin Nutr 62:1–9, 1995

Hibbeln JR, Umhau J, George D, et al: Do plasma polyunsaturates predict hostility and depression? World Rev Nutr Diet 82:175–186, 1997

Hobbs C, Amster M: Naturopathic specific condition review: premenstrual syndrome. Professional Journal of Botanical Medicine, Spring 1996, pp 168–173

Horton R: Benign prostatic hyperplasia: a disorder of the androgen metabolism in the male. J Am Geriatr Soc 32:380–385, 1984

Ianiello A, Ostuni PA, Sfriso P, et al: *S*-Adenosyl-L-methionine in Sjögren's syndrome and fibromyalgia. Current Therapeutic Research, Clinical and Experimental 55:699–705, 1994

Jacobsen FM: Fluoxetine-induced sexual dysfunction and an open trial of yohimbine. J Clin Psychiatry 53:119–122, 1992

Jacobsen S, Danneskiold-Samsoe B, Andersen RB: Oral *S*-adenosylmethionine in primary fibromyalgia: double-blind clinical evaluation. Scand J Rheumatol 20:294–302, 1991

Jamieson DD, Duffield PH: The antinociceptive actions of kava components in mice. Clin Exp Pharmacol Physiol 17:495–507, 1990

Jan JE, Espezel H, Appleton RE: The treatment of sleep disorders with melatonin. Dev Med Child Neurol 36:97–107, 1994

Janicak PG, Lipinski J, Davis J, et al: *S*-Adenosylmethionine in depression: a literature review and preliminary report. Ala J Med Sci 25:306–313, 1988

Jellin JM, Batz F, Hitchens K: Pharmacist's Letter/Prescriber's Letter Natural Medicines Comprehensive Database. Stockton, CA, Therapeutic Research Faculty, 1999

Jensen CL, Chen H, Fraley JK, et al: Biochemical affects of dietary linoleic/alpha-linolenic acid ratio in term infants. Lipids 31:107–113, 1996

Jorgensen HM, Hernell O, Lund P, et al: Visual acuity and erythrocyte docosahexanoic acid status in breast-fed and formula-fed term infants during the first four months of life. Lipids 31:99–105, 1996

Kagan BL, Sultzer DL, Rosenlicht N, et al: Oral *S*-adenosylmethionine in depression: a randomized, double-blind, placebo-controlled trial. Am J Psychiatry 147:591–595, 1990

Kang SY, Kim SH, Schini VB, et al: Dietary ginsenosides improve endothelium-dependent relaxation in the thoracic aorta of hypercholesterolemic rabbit. Gen Pharmacol 26:483–487, 1995

Kasper S: Treatment of seasonal affective disorder (SAD) with hypericum extract. Pharmacopsychiatry 30(suppl 2):89–93, 1997

Keville K: Red clover. Better Nutrition, March 1999, p 34

Kleijnen J, Ter Riet G, Knaipschild P: Vitamin B_6 in the treatment of premenstrual syndrome—a review. Br J Obstet Gynaecol 97:847–852, 1990

Klepser T, Nisly N: Chaste tree berry for premenstrual syndrome. Alternative Medicine Alert 2(6):61–72, 1999

Ko RJ: Adulterants in Asian patent medicines (letter). N Engl J Med 339:847, 1998

Konig H, Stahl H, Sleper J, et al: Magnetic resonance tomography of finger polyarthritis: morphology and cartilage signals after ademetionine therapy. Aktuelle Radiol 5:36–40, 1995

Kowluru A, Rana S, MacDonald MJ: Phospholipid methyltransferase activity in pancreatic islets: activation by calcium. Arch Biochem Biophys 242(1):72–81, 1985

Kowluru A, Seavey SE, Rabaglia ME, et al: Carboxylmethylation of the catalytic subunit of protein phosphatase 2A in insulin-secreting cells: evidence for functional consequences on enzyme activity and insulin secretion. Endocrinology 137(6):2315–2323, 1996

Krzeski T, Kazon M, Borkowski A, et al: Combined extracts of *Urtica dioca* and *Pygeum africanum* in the treatment of benign prostatic hyperplasia: double-blind comparison of two doses. Clin Ther 15:1011–1020, 1993

Kunz D, Bes F: Melatonin effects in a patient with severe REM sleep behavior disorder: case report and theoretical considerations. Neuropsychobiology 36:211–214, 1997

Kyle DJ, Schaefer E, Patton G, et al: Low serum docosahexanoic acid is a significant risk factor for Alzheimer's dementia. Presentation at the 3rd ISSFAL Congress, Lyons, France, June 1–5, 1998

Laakmann G, Schule C, Baghai T, et al: St. John's Wort in mild to moderate depression: the relevance of hyperforin for the clinical efficacy. Pharmacopsychiatry 31(suppl 1):54–59, 1998

Laraki L, Pelletier X, Mourot J, et al: Effects of dietary phytosterols on liver, lipids and lipid metabolism enzymes. Ann Nutr Metab 37:129–133, 1993

Lauritzen C, Reuter HD, Repges R, et al: Treatment of premenstrual tension syndrome with *Vitex agnus castus*: controlled, double-blind study versus pyridoxine. Phytomedicine 4:183–189, 1997

Lehmann E, Kinzler E, Friedmann J, et al: Efficacy of a special kava extract (*Piper methysticum*) in patients with states of anxiety, tension, excitedness of non-mental origin—a double-blind, placebo-controlled study of four weeks treatment. Phytomedicine 3:113–119, 1996

Levine J, Barak Y, Gonzalves M, et al: Double-blind, controlled trial of inositol treatment of depression. Am J Psychiatry 152:792–794, 1995

Lichius JJ, Muth C: The inhibiting effects of *Urtica dioica* root extracts on experimentally induced prostatic hyperplasia in the mouse. Planta Med 63:307–310, 1997

Lieberman S: Nutriceutical review of St. John's wort (*Hypericum perforatum*) for the treatment of depression. J Womens Health 7:177–182, 1998a

Lieberman S: A review of the effectiveness of *Cimicifuga racemosa* (Black cohosh) for the symptoms of menopause. J Womens Health 7:525–559, 1998b

Liebman B: The soy story. Nutrition Action Newsletter, September 1998, pp 3–7

Lightfoote J, Blair J, Cohen JR: Lead intoxication in an adult caused by Chinese herbal medication. JAMA 238:1539, 1977

Linde K, Ramirez G, Mulrow CD, et al: St. John's wort for depression—an overview and meta-analysis of randomised clinical trials. BMJ 313:253–258, 1996

Lindenberg D, Pitule-Schodel HD: D,L-Kavain in comparison with oxazepam and anxiety disorders: a double-blind study of clinical effectiveness. Fortschr Med 108:49–50, 53–54, 1990

Lock M: Contested meanings of menopause. Lancet 337:1270–1272, 1991

Loehrer FM, Angst CP, Haefeli WE, et al: Low whole-blood S-adenosyl-methionine and correlation between 5-methyltetrahydrofolate and homocysteine in coronary artery disease. Arterioscler Thromb Vasc Biol 16:727–733, 1996

Loehrer FM, Schwab R, Angst CP, et al: Influence of oral S-adenosylmethionine on plasma 5-methyltetrahydrofolate, S-adenosylhomocysteine, homocysteine and methionine in healthy humans. J Pharmacol Exp Ther 282:845–850, 1997

Lolic MM, Fiskum G, Rosenthal RE: Neuroprotective effects of acetyl-L-carnitine after stroke in rats. Ann Emerg Med 29:758–765, 1997

Lonnrot K, Porsti I, Alho H, et al: Control of arterial tone after long-term coenzyme Q10 supplementation in senescent rats. Br J Pharmacol 124:1500–1506, 1998

Maes M: Fatty acids, cytokines, and major depression (editorial). Biol Psychiatry 42:313–314, 1998

Maggioni M, Picotti GB, Bondiolotti GP, et al: Effects of phosphatidylserine therapy in geriatric patients with depressive disorders. Acta Psychiatr Scand 81:265–270, 1990

Makrides M, Neumann MA, Gibson RA: Is dietary docosahexanoic acid essential for term infants? Lipids 31:115–119, 1996

Mangoni A, Grassi MP, Frattola L, et al: Effects of a MAO-B inhibitor in the treatment of Alzheimer disease. Eur Neurol 31(2):100–107, 1991

Martinez B, Lipinski JK, Kasper S, et al: Hypericum in the treatment of seasonal affective disorder. J Geriatr Psychiatry Neurol 7(suppl 1):S29–S33, 1994

Mathews JD, Riley MD, Fego J, et al: Effects of the heavy usage of kava on physical health: summary of a pilot survey in an Aboriginal community. Med J Aust 148:548–555, 1988

Mayo JL: A natural approach to menopause. Clinical Nutrition Insights 5(7):1–8, 1997

McCaleb R: Vitex Agnus-Castus. Golden, CO, Herb Research Foundation, May 1995

McLeod MN, Gaynes BN, Golden RN: Chromium potentiation of antidepressant pharmacotherapy for dysthymic disorder in five patients. J Clin Psychiatry 60:237–240, 1999

Meeker JE, Reynolds PC: Postmortem tissue methamphetamine concentrations following seligiline administration. J Anal Toxicol 14:330–331, 1990

Melatonin. The Medical Letter 37:111, 1995

Milkiewicz P, Mills CO, Roma MG, et al: Tauroursodeoxycholate and *S*-adenosyl-L-methionine exert an additive ameliorating effect on tau-rolithocholate-induced cholestatis: a study in isolated rat hepatocyte couplets. Hepatology 29:471–476, 1999

Miller LG: Herbal medicinals: selected clinical considerations focusing on known or potential drug-herb interactions. Arch Intern Med 158:2200–2211, 1998

Morales A, Condra M, Owen J, et al: Is yohimbine effective in the treatment of organic impotence? Results of a controlled trial. J Urol 137:1168–1172, 1987

Morrison LD, Smith DD, Kish SJ: Brain *S*-adenosylmethionine levels are severely decreased in Alzheimer's disease. J Neurochem 67:1328–1331, 1996

Mowrey DB: Muira-Puama (Liriosma ovata), in Herbal Tonic Therapies. Avenel, NJ, Wings Books, 1996, pp 305–359

Muller WE, Rolli M, Schafer C, et al: Effects of hypericum extract in biochemical models of antidepressant activity. Pharmacopsychiatry 30:102–107, 1997

Muller WE, Singer A, Wonnemann M, et al: Hyperforin represents the neurotransmitter reuptake inhibiting constituent of hypericum extract. Pharmacopsychiatry 31(suppl):16–21, 1998

Nidecker A: Probing genes, drugs, and fatty acids in dementia. Clinical Psychiatry News, December 1997, p 4

Otero-Losada ME, Rubio MC: Acute changes in 5-HT metabolism after *S*-adenosylmethionine administration. Gen Pharmacol 20:403–406, 1989a

Otero-Losada ME, Rubio MC: Acute effects of *S*-adenosyl-L-methionine on catecholaminergic central function. Eur J Pharmacol 163:353–356, 1989b

Packer L, Colman C: The Antioxidant Miracle. New York, Wiley, 1999

Palevitch D, Earon G, Carasso R: Feverfew as a prophylactic treatment for migraine: a double-blind placebo-controlled study. Phytother Res 11:506–511, 1997

Parry BL: A 45-year-old woman with premenstrual dysphoric disorder. JAMA 281:368–373, 1999

Peet M, Murphy B, Shay J, et al: Depletion of omega-3 fatty acid levels in red blood cell membranes of depressive patients. Biol Psychiatry 43:315–319, 1998

Pepeu G, Pepeu IM, Amaducci L: A review of phosphatidylserine pharmacological and clinical effects: is phosphatidylserine a drug for the aging brain? Pharmacol Res 33(2):73–80, 1996

Pezzoli C, Galli-Kienle M, Stramentinoli G: Lack of mutagenic activity of ademetionine in vitro and in vivo. Arzneimittelforschung 37:826–829, 1987

Quiros CF, Cardenas RA: Maca (Lepidium meyenii Walp.), in Andean Roots and Tubers: Ahipa, Arracacha, Maca, Yacon. Promoting the Conservation and Use of Underutilized and Neglected Crops, Vol 21. Edited by Herman M, Heller J. Rome, Italy, Institute of Plant Genetics and Crop Plant Research, Gatersleben/International Plant Resources Institute, 1997, pp 184–185

Rako S: Testosterone deficiency and supplementation for women: matters of sexuality and health. Psychiatric Annals 29:23–26, 1999

Raloff J: Does life have a dark side? Nighttime illumination might elevate cancer risk. Science News 154:248–250, 1998

Ramsey JJ, Colman RJ, Swick AG, et al: Energy expenditure, body composition, and glucose metabolism in lean and obese rhesus monkeys treated with ephedrine and caffeine. Am J Clin Nutr 68:42–51, 1998

Rau AV, Janezic SA: The role of dietary phytosterols in colon carcinogenesis. Nutr Cancer 18:43–51, 1992

Reiter RJ: Melatonin. New York, Bantam, 1996

Reynolds EH, Camey MWP, Toone BK, et al: Transmethylation and neuropsychiatry, in Biochemical, Pharmacological, and Clinical Aspects of Transmethylation. Edited by Mato J. Cell Biology Reviews 2:93–100, 1987

Reynolds EH, Godfrey P, Bottiglieri T, et al: S-Adenosylmethionine and Alzheimer's disease (abstract). Neurology 39:397, 1989

Robbers JE, Tyler VE: Tyler's Herbs of Choice: The Therapeutic Use of Phytomedicinals. New York, Hawthorne Herbal Press, 1999

Rosenbaum JF, Fava M, Falk WE, et al: The antidepressant potential of oral S-adenosyl-L-methionine. Acta Psychiatr Scand 81:432–436, 1990

Rosenfeld FL, Pepe S, Ou R, et al: Coenzyme Q10 improves the tolerance of the senescent myocardium to aerobic and ischemic stress: studies in rats and in human atrial tissue. Biofactors 9(2–4):291–299, 1999

Saklad SR: Patients with schizophrenia have decreased RBC membrane fatty acids. Psychopharmacology Update 9(12):1–7, 1998

Salem N Jr: Omega-3 fatty acids: molecular and biochemical aspects, in New Roles for Selective Nutrients. Edited by Spiller GA, Scala J. New York, Alan R Liss, 1989, pp 109–228

Salem N Jr, Kim HY, Yergey JA: Docosohexanoic acid: membrane function and metabolism, in Health Effects of Polyunsaturated Seafoods, Vol 15. Edited by Simopoulos A, Kifer RR, Martin R. New York, Academic Press, 1986, pp 263–317

Salmaggi P, Bressa GM, Nicchia G, et al: Double-blind, placebo-controlled study of S-adenosylmethionine in depressed postmenopausal women. Psychother Psychosom 59:34–40, 1993

Sayegh R, Schiff I, Wurtman J, et al: The effect of a carbohydrate-rich beverage on mood, appetite, and cognitive function in women with premenstrual syndrome. Obstet Gynecol 86:520–528, 1995

Schaumburg HH, Berger A: Alopecia and sensory polyneuropathy from thallium in a Chinese herbal medication. JAMA 268:3430–3431, 1992

Schellenberg R, Sauer S, Dimpfel W: Pharmacodynamic effects of two different hypericum extracts in healthy volunteers measured by quantitative EEG. Pharmacopsychiatry 31:44–53, 1998

Schenck CH, Bundlie SR, Ettinger MG, et al: Chronic behavioral disorders of human REM sleep: a new category of parasomnia. Sleep 9:293–308, 1986

Schultz V, Hubner WD, Ploch M: Clinical trials with phytopsychopharmacological agents. Phytomedicine 4:379–387, 1997

Shekim WO, Antun F, Hanna G, et al: S-Adenosyl-L-methionine (SAM) in adults with ADHD: preliminary results from an open trial. Psychopharmacol Bull 26:249–253, 1990

Simons AJ, Dawson IK, Duguma B, et al: Passing problems: prostate and prunus. Herbalgram 43:49–53, 1998

Simopoulos AP: Omega-3 fatty acids in health and disease and in growth and development. Am J Clin Nutr 54:438–463, 1991

Singh NN, Ellis CR, Singh YN: A double-blind, placebo-controlled study of the effects of kava (Kavatrol) on daily stress and anxiety in adults. Alternative Therapies in Health and Medicine 4(2):97–98, 1998

Singh YN, Blumenthal M: Kava: an overview. Herbalgram 39:33–55, 1996

Skolnick AW: Scientific verdict still out on DHEA. Medical News and Perspectives. JAMA 276:1365–1367, 1996

Soderberg M, Edlund C, Kristensson K, et al: Fatty acid composition of brain phospholipids in aging and in Alzheimer's disease. Lipids 26:421–425, 1991

Soffa VM: Alternatives to hormone replacement for menopause. Alternative Therapies 2(2):34–39, 1996

Sohn M, Sikora R: Ginkgo biloba extract in the therapy of erectile dysfunction. Journal of Sex Education Therapy 17:53–61, 1991

Sorenson H, Sonne J: A double-masked study of the effects of ginseng on cognitive functions. Current Therapeutic Research, Clinical and Experimental 57:959–968, 1996

Sotaniemi EA, Haapakoski E, Rautio A: Ginseng therapy in non–insulin-dependent diabetic patients. Diabetes Care 18:1373–1375, 1995

Steinberg S, Annable L, Young SN, et al: A placebo-controlled clinical trial of L-tryptophan in premenstrual dysphoria. Biol Psychiatry 45:313–320, 1999

Stevens LJ, Zentall SS, Deck JL, et al: Essential fatty acid metabolism in boys with attention defecit hyperactivity disorder. Am J Clin Nutr 62:761–768, 1995

Stoll AL, Sachs GS, Cohen BM, et al: Choline in the treatment of rapid-cycling bipolar disorder: clinical and neurochemical findings in lithium-treated patients. Biol Psychiatry 40:382–388, 1996

Stoll AL, Severus WE, Freeman MP, et al: Omega-3 fatty acids in bipolar disorder: a preliminary double-blind, placebo-controlled trial. Arch Gen Psychiatry 56:407–412, 1999

Stramentinoli G: Pharmacologic aspects of S-adenosylmethionine: pharmacokinetics and pharmacodynamics. Am J Med 83(5A):35–42, 1987

Surtees R, Hyland K: A method for the measurement of S-adenosylmethionine in small volumes of cerebrospinal fluid or brain using high performance liquid chromatography-electrochemistry. Anal Biochem 181:331–335, 1989

Tavoni A, Vitali C, Bombardieri S, et al: Evaluation of S-adenosylmethionine in primary fibromyalgia: a double-blind crossover study. Am J Med 83(5A):107–110, 1987

Tavoni A, Jeracitano G, Cirigliano G: Evaluation of S-adenosylmethionine in secondary fibromyalgia: a double-blind study (letter). Clin Exp Rheumatol 16:106–107, 1998

Taylor KM, Randall PK: Depletion of S-adenosyl-L-methionine in mouse brain by antidepressive drugs. J Pharmacol Exp Ther 194:303–310, 1975

Teufel-Mayer R, Gleitz J: Effects of long-term administration of hypericum extracts on affinity and density of the central serotonergic 5-HT$_{1A}$ and 5-HT$_{2A}$ receptors. Pharmacopsychiatry 30:113–116, 1997

Thiele B, Brink I, Ploch M: Modulation of cytokine expression by hypericum extract. J Geriatr Psychiatry Neurol 7(suppl 1):S60–S62, 1994

Thommessen B, Laake K: No identifiable effect of ginseng (Gericomplex) as an adjuvant in the treatment of geriatric patients. Aging Clin Exp Res 8:417–420, 1996

Thys-Jacobs S, Ceccarelli S, Bierman A, et al: Calcium supplementation in premenstrual syndrome: a randomized, crossover study. J Gen Intern Med 4:183–189, 1989

Thys-Jacobs S, Starkey P, Bernstein D, et al: Calcium carbonate and the premenstrual sydrome: effects on premenstrual and menstrual symptoms. Am J Obstet Gynecol 179:444–452, 1998

Toffano G, Leon A, Benvegnu D, et al: Effect of brain phospholipids on the catecholamine content of mouse brain. Pharmacol Res Commun 8:581–590, 1976

Torta R, Zanalda F, Rocca P, et al: Inhibitory activity of S-adenosyl-L-methionine on serum gamma-glutamyl-transpeptidase increase induced by psychodrugs and anticonvulsants. Current Therapeutic Research, Clinical and Experimental 44:144–159, 1988

Toubro S, Astrup A, Breum L, et al: The acute and chronic effects of ephedrine/caffeine mixtures on energy expenditure and glucose metabolism in humans. Int J Obes Relat Metab Disord 17(suppl 3):S73–S77, 1993

Turyn D, Scacchi GE, Dellacha JM: Unmasking of insulin receptors in rat submaxillary gland microsomes: effect of high ionic strength, phospholipase C, and S-adenosylmethonine. Biochem Biophys Acta 845(3):333–342, 1985

Uchida K, Mizuno H, Hirota K, et al: Effects of spinasterol and sitosterol on plasma and liver cholesterol levels and biliary and fecal sterol and bile acid excretions in mice. Jpn J Pharmacol 33:103–112, 1983

Voelker R: Herbs and anesthesia. JAMA 281:1882, 1999

Volkmann H, Norregaard J, Jacobsen S, et al: Double-blind, placebo-controlled cross-over study of intravenous S-adenosyl-L-methionine in patients with fibromyalgia. Scand J Rheumatol 26:206–211, 1997

Volz HP, Kieser M: Kava-kava extract WS 1490 versus placebo in anxiety disorders—a randomized placebo-controlled 25 week outpatient trial. Pharmacopsychiatry 30:1–5, 1997

Vorbach EU, Arnoldt KH, Hubner WD: Efficacy and tolerability of St. John's wort extract, LI 160, versus imipramine in patients with severe depressive episodes according to ICD-10. Pharmacopsychiatry 30:81–85, 1997

Warnecke G: Psychosomatic dysfunctions in the female climacteric: clinical effectiveness and tolerance of kava extract [in German]. Fortschr Med 109(4):119–122, 1991

Waynberg J: Aphrodisiacs: contribution to the clinical validation of the traditional use of Ptychopetalum guyanna. Presentation at the First International Congress on Ethnopharmacology, Strasbourg, France, June 5–9, 1990

Werner P, DiRocco A, Rempel T, et al: COMT-dependent protection of dopamine neurons against L-dopa toxicity by methionine, dimethionine, and S-adenosylmethionine. J Neurochem 73(suppl):S10C, 1999

Wesnes KA, Faleni RA, Hefting NR, et al: The cognitive subjective and physical effects of a *Ginkgo biloba–Panax ginseng* combination in healthy volunteers with neurasthenic complaints. Psychopharmacol Bull 33:677–683, 1997

Wheatley D: Li 160, an extract of St. John's Wort, versus amitriptyline in mildly to moderately-depressed outpatients—a controlled 6-week clinical trial. Pharmacopsychiatry 30:77–80, 1997

Wheatley D: Hypericum in seasonal affective disorder (SAD). Curr Med Res Opin 15:33–37, 1999

Willats P, Forsyth JS, DiModugno MK, et al: Effect of long-chain polyunsaturated fatty acids in infant formula on problem solving at 10 months of age. Lancet 352:688–691, 1998

Wilt TJ, Ushani A, Stark G, et al: Saw palmetto extracts for treatment of benign prostatic hyperplasia: a systematic review. JAMA 280:1604–1609, 1998

Witte VB, Harrer G, Kaptan T, et al: Treatment of depressive symptoms with a high concentration hypericum preparation: a multicenter, placebo-controlled, double-blind study. Fortschr Med 113(28):404–408, 1995

Wolkowitz O, Reus V, Keebler A, et al: Double-blind treatment of major depression with dehydroepiandrosterone. Am J Psychiatry 156:646–649, 1999

Wong AHC, Smith M, Boon HS: Herbal remedies in psychiatric practice. Arch Gen Psychiatry 55:1033–1034, 1998

Yager J, Siegfreid SL, DiMatteo TL: Use of alternative remedies by psychiatric patients: illustrative vignettes and a discussion of the issues. Am J Psychiatry 156:1432–1438, 1999

Chapter 2

Acupuncture for Mental Health

Francine Rainone, D.O.

If Qi and Blood exist in abundance and harmony, a person will not get sick. Once there is depression, all kinds of diseases will start to evolve. Therefore all of the body's diseases are caused by depression.

Zhu Danxi

There is no mental illness in traditional Chinese medicine (TCM). The phenomena that Westerners call anxiety, depression, and psychosis create suffering in China, as they do throughout the world. However, the conceptual framework of TCM neither isolates soma, psyche, and soul nor severs human beings from each other and the natural world to center its views of health around the individual. My discussion of using acupuncture for "psychiatric disorders" begins with an exploration of the TCM view of the world, the place of humans in it, and the processes of health and disease. Then I briefly review the scientific hypotheses for the efficacy of acupuncture and, finally, discuss the research, indications, and cautions regarding the contemporary use of acupuncture for so-called mental illnesses.

This review is limited in several ways. It focuses on the Chinese approach. The literature searched is almost exclusively in English, whereas the bulk of research activity in this area is published in Chinese and Japanese. And as in any vibrant tradition, there is not unanimity on these topics among practitioners of TCM. I have downplayed the disagreements in the interest of presenting a lu-

---

It is my pleasure to thank Mindy Fullilove, Dan Bensky, and Fumiyo Akazawa for support and challenging critiques of the manuscript and David Walker for invaluable editorial assistance in its preparation.

cid, readable introduction to this topic. Technical terms in Chinese medicine are capitalized to distinguish them from their meanings in common English; for example, Cold is a pathogenic factor in TCM rather than a relative temperature, and the Liver is a complex set of functions in the body rather than simply a specific bodily tissue. Despite these limitations I hope this review will provide a conceptual framework for appreciating acupuncture from the perspective of a rigorous intellectual tradition several millennia older than our own.

Overview of Traditional Chinese Medicine

Fundamental Theories of Traditional Chinese Medicine

TCM is based on the twin pillars of *Yin-Yang theory* and *Five Phase theory*. Yin-Yang theory is older and more empirically based, and the two theories do not always yield the same conclusions about etiology, pathophysiology, or treatment of disease. Some schools emphasize one theory or the other, but they are both used to some extent by all TCM practitioners. Rather than being a source of conflict or incoherence, this tension works to add depth and flexibility to clinical practice. TCM is incomprehensible without at least a passing understanding of these theories.

Yin-Yang Theory

Yin-Yang theory has its origins in Taoism and the earliest roots of Chinese culture. A global theory, it is meant to explain everything in the universe. There are five basic tenets to the theory, all of which are expressed by the Taoist symbol reproduced in Figure 2–1. (The following discussion is based on Kaptchuk 1983, pp. 8–11.)

1. Everything in the universe is fundamentally composed of a Yin aspect and a Yang aspect. Accordingly, the circle is divided into black (representing Yin) and white (representing Yang) parts.
2. Every Yin aspect has a Yang aspect and every Yang aspect has a Yin aspect. This is why the black portion of the whole includes a white circle and the white portion includes a black circle.

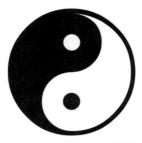

Figure 2–1. The Yin-Yang symbol (Taiji).
Source. From *Acupuncture: A Comprehensive Text* by the Shanghai College of Traditional Medicine, translated and edited by John O'Connor and Dan Bensky, with permission of Eastland Press, P.O. Box 99749, Seattle, WA 98199. Copyright 1981. All rights reserved.

3. Yin and Yang mutually create each other.
4. Yin and Yang balance (control) each other in a homeostatic fashion.

   The third and fourth tenets are expressed by the fact that the Yin portion extends into the Yang part of the circle and the Yang portion extends into the Yin part, and the fact that equal portions of the circle are one or the other color, but their respective territories are not neatly divided in two.
5. Yin and Yang transform into each other. The curving of the line delineating the two areas expresses this dynamism.

Yin-Yang theory establishes several fundamental principles about the nature of reality. First, reality is relational. Nothing (and no one) in the universe exists or can be understood except in relation to everything else. Every duality is a unity of opposites that exists in continuity on a continuum. Second, the universe is continuously changing, as Yin and Yang create, balance, and transform into each other. Third, this change proceeds according to patterns determined by the nature of Yin and Yang. The universe, however diverse it appears, is a unity whose mechanisms function to preserve overall homeostasis. In this sense, the earliest beginnings of ecologic thinking are arguably within early Chinese thought. Using the theory of Yin and Yang, the wise person can make sense of the most confusing situation, can predict what will happen if natural processes are left to their own development, and can skillfully intervene to alter the outcome. As in any other field, these fundamental principles are not subject to question or examination, but rather form the framework in which questions about reality are asked and answered.

Applied to medicine, Yin-Yang theory guided the development of thousands of years of empirical observations into a phenomenology of health and disease. Because there is no separation of humans from the environment, the workings of the natural world and the human body are governed by the same principles and subject to the same sorts of disturbance. This idea is clearly expressed by the concept of the six Excesses, or Pernicious Influences, which are Wind, Heat, Cold, Dampness, Dryness, and Summer Heat. When normal forces in the environment become excessive or occur out of season, the balance of Yin and Yang is disturbed. In the struggle to restore balance there may be natural or human disasters. For example, just as unchecked growth in forests generates fires, excess Heat in the body can be damaging. Sometimes a forest fire restores homeostasis in the ecologic system in which it occurs. At other times it destroys all or part of that system. Similarly, someone exposed to Cold (a Yin condition) may subsequently develop Heat in the form of a fever (a Yang condition created by the Yin). If the Heat is intense enough to control the Cold, the body returns to balance. If the Heat rages out of control, the person may go into shock and become quite cold to the touch (transformation of Yang into Yin, of Heat into Cold). Illness in Yin-Yang theory is a disturbance of homeostasis. It is described in terms of observable events and processes of and in the person. Notice that the struggle to regain homeostasis depends on two factors: the strength of the Excess and the strength of the system it disturbs. Not all trees fall in a hurricane, and not all people break bones when they fall or become infected with pneumonia after exposure.

So what is Cold? To begin with, Cold is a subjective feeling of decreased temperature or a state of feeling cold to the touch. Just as Cold can freeze the environment, it can cause contraction and stiffness in the body, which may be painful. Watery clear secretions, an aversion to cold temperatures, and a desire for warmth are also characteristic of Cold disharmonies. Notice that Cold does not cause disease. The strength of TCM is phenomenology, not etiology; it describes patterns of change in the body in terms of human experience. Someone with a high fever who has chills is suffering from Cold, not Heat. Cold is not *the cause* of the disease; it *is* the disease (see Kaptchuk 1983, pp. 115–137). In Western medicine, decisions about treatment are hindered in the absence of a known cause. In TCM, what you see is what you treat. The pattern in a particular person is the disease process.

Five Phase Theory

Unfortunately, certain English translations of acupuncture texts render "Wu Xing" as "Five Elements" rather than Five Phases. (The following discussion is based on Kaptchuk 1983, pp. 343–357.) This leads to the belief that early TCM resembled the Greek theory that everything in the world could be broken down into four basic constituent parts—Air, Earth, Fire, and Water—and later European medical theories based on the "humors." Nothing could be further from the truth. *Wu* is Chinese for the number five, and *Xing* means walk or move. Thus, the Five Phases are processes or properties, not constituents. They are meant to explain the dynamics of relationships.

The Phases are denoted Wood, Fire, Earth, Metal, and Water. Each Phase is associated with a wide variety of phenomena, including season, color, emotion, direction, sound, Organ, tissue, orifice, taste, and smell (Table 2–1). Rather than being inductions based on observation, the Phases arrange sets of observable phenomena around images suggested by a metaphysical understanding of the process of growth and decay. For example, the Wood phase is associated with spring and things that are in the active process of growing and developing. Fire represents summer and a state of maximal activity about to decline or enter dormancy. Metal represents autumn and processes of decline. Water represents winter and the maximal state of rest, whereas Earth represents the transition between seasons (and often designates Indian summer) and balance or neutrality.

The Phases can be related to one another in many ways, but the two patterns with the most effect on medical practice are the Producing and Controlling (or Conquest) cycles (Figure 2–2). In the

Table 2–1. Correspondences associated with the five phases

	Wood	Fire	Earth	Metal	Water
Direction	East	South	Center	West	North
Season	Spring	Summer	Long Summer	Autumn	Winter
Climatic condition	Wind	Summer heat	Dampness	Dryness	Cold
Process	Birth	Growth	Transformation	Harvest	Storage
Color	Green	Red	Yellow	White	Black
Taste	Sour	Bitter	Sweet	Pungent	Salty
Smell	Goatish	Burning	Fragrant	Rank	Rotten
Yin organ	Liver	Heart	Spleen	Lungs	Kidneys
Yang organ	Gall bladder	Small intestine	Stomach	Large intestine	Bladder
Opening	Eyes	Tongue	Mouth	Nose	Ears
Tissue	Sinews	Blood vessels	Flesh	Skin/Hair	Bones
Emotion	Anger	Happiness	Pensiveness	Sadness	Fear
Human sound	Shout	Laughter	Song	Weeping	Groan

Source. From *Acupuncture: A Comprehensive Text* by the Shanghai College of Traditional Medicine, translated and edited by John O'Connor and Dan Bensky, with permission of Eastland Press, P.O. Box 99749, Seattle, WA 98199. Copyright 1981. All rights reserved.

Producing cycle, Wood produces Fire that produces Earth that produces Metal that produces Water that produces Wood. This cycle is clinically useful in explaining Deficiency patterns and choosing treatments for them. The Producer is referred to as the Mother, and the Produced is referred to as the Child. The Child of a Deficient Mother may itself become Deficient from lack of nourishment. Or if a Child is Deficient it may drain the Mother, making it Deficient as well. Thus, if the Liver (Wood) is deficient, it can be treated by strengthening the Kidneys (Water). If the Heart (Fire) is in Excess, it can be treated by draining the Spleen (Earth). Disharmonies of the control cycle are similarly useful clinically. One Organ may overcontrol another, leading to Deficiency in one or both of them, or the Organ that should be controlled may become the controller, leading to an excess or deficiency in that Organ.

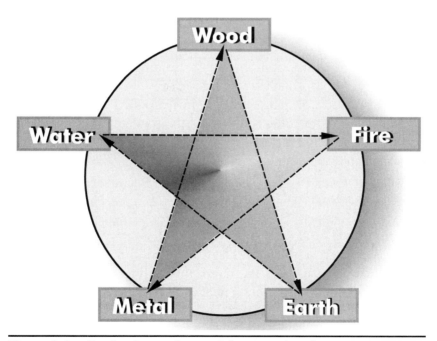

Figure 2–2. Production and control (conquest) cycles.
Source. From *Acupuncture: A Comprehensive Text* by the Shanghai College of Traditional Medicine, translated and edited by John O'Connor and Dan Bensky, with permission of Eastland Press, P.O. Box 99749, Seattle, WA 98199. Copyright 1981. All rights reserved.

Pathophysiology

Pathophysiology in TCM is based on an understanding of the Vital Substances, the Organs, and the Channels. I discuss three of the five Vital Substances: Qi, Jing, and Shen, which are called the Three Treasures. Note that what we translate as "substances" are not just different types of stuff; they are conceptualized and understood in terms of their *functions* in the body (see Kaptchuk 1983, pp. 34–49).

Vital Substances

The Three Treasures

Despite popular beliefs, Qi is not "energy." Nor is it matter. Some of the functions of Qi are more material, some are more energetic. In TCM, this poses no problems, because matter and energy, like all dualities, are on a continuum. *Qi* is the source of all motion and action in the body; it protects the body, is the source of transformation in the body, is responsible for holding all substances and Organs in their proper place, and warms the body. *Jing* is the source of life and of instinctual organic processes. Prenatal Jing, or congenital essence, is roughly equivalent to genetic endowment. Postnatal Jing is derived from food. Together they provide the substrate that enables individuals to grow, develop, and reproduce.

Shen has been translated in two main ways, neither of which is entirely satisfactory. If translated as Spirit, the impression is given that it is nonmaterial and persists after death. If translated as Mind, it becomes too closely associated with the brain and thinking. Neither translation captures its materiality, which is crucial to the TCM understanding of mental health. Shen is closest to that awkward rubric Body–Mind–Spirit. In what follows, I have chosen not to translate it. The simplest expression of the materiality of the Shen is the belief that both parents contribute to the Shen before birth, but that it also is continually, literally nourished after birth. Diet, physical activity, emotions, sexual activity, and drugs all affect the Shen. In one meaning of the word (Maciocia 1994, pp. 197–199), Shen encompasses all mental activities and characteristics, including thinking, consciousness, insight, intelligence, cognition, wisdom, formation of ideas, sleep, and memory.

None of these three substances can be deeply understood without understanding the others. Qi helps transform food into post-natal Jing, but without prenatal Jing there could be no life or Qi. Many references say that the Jing of the mother and father come together to form the Shen of the child. "If [Jing] is strong, Qi flourishes; if Qi flourishes[,] the [Shen] is whole" (*Zhang Jie Bin* 1624/1982, cited in Maciocia 1994, p. 198).

The main point about the Vital Substances is their dynamism. They are constantly created, transformed, and circulated throughout the body. Anything that drains or fails to supply the necessities for their creation, disturbs their transformation, or impedes their circulation disrupts the homeostasis of the individual. One can regard Jing as the densest form of Qi and Shen as the most refined form of Qi. Thus, anything that affects the Qi can disturb the Shen or deplete the body's store of Jing, which in turn will disturb the Shen.

The Organs

The Vital Substances are created, transformed, and circulated in and through a system of Organs. There are 12 major Organs, grouped into six pairs of one Yin and one Yang Organ. The five major Yin Organs are the Heart, Lungs, Spleen, Liver, and Kidneys. They are of more importance to medical theory because they produce, transform, regulate, and store the Vital Substances. In particular, the Heart stores the Shen, the Lungs and Spleen produce the Qi, the Liver guides the harmonious flow of Qi through the body, and the Kidneys store the Jing.

Unlike Western anatomy, which identifies organs as gross physical structures, in TCM, Organs are (almost) all associated with a bodily tissue but never reducible to it; Organs are defined by what they "do." Perhaps in part because they did not begin reasoning from the physical structure, Chinese medical practitioners were free to correlate their observations into functional units. Now it is "common sense" to observe that the kidneys affect respiration, but before the complex system for regulating bicarbonate was understood this would have been regarded as madness. In TCM, for thousands of years it has been a truism that the Kidneys "complete the breath."

The Channels

The Organs are interconnected by a system of Channels that traverse the body and allow communication and transportation among the Organs. (Because meridians are two-dimensional, that term does not capture the transporting function that is essential to the Channels.) Acupuncture points are locations on the Channels where communication and transportation can be regulated (Figure 2–3). In a commonly employed metaphor, the Channels are compared to the electrical wiring in a building; the acupuncture points to light switches, dimmers, and fuses; and the Organs to appliances. In this room, electricity (the Vital Substances) "becomes" images on television. In the next room, it cooks dinner and washes the dishes. Everywhere it provides light. TCM considers the "depth" of the disturbance to be of prime importance to its treatment. In general, the surface of the body and the Channels are more exterior. A Pernicious Influence may enter the body and be successfully repelled at the level of the Channels, or it may travel through the Channels into the Organs. From one Organ it may travel through Channels to other Organs. For example, Liver Wind may travel through the Liver Channel to the head, manifesting as dizziness, or may enter other Channels, manifesting as numbness or tremors in the limbs. In addition, Organs are considered in terms of their relative depth. The Lungs are less interior and the Kidneys are relatively deep, so the Lungs are often the first Organs to be attacked by external influences.

Categories of Disease Process

Disease processes can all be grouped into three categories: those that deplete or interrupt the production of Vital Substances, which commonly results in Deficiency; those that interfere with transformation, which commonly results in accumulation of Excess; and those that impede circulation, which commonly results in Stagnation. Usually these processes interact, and the develop-

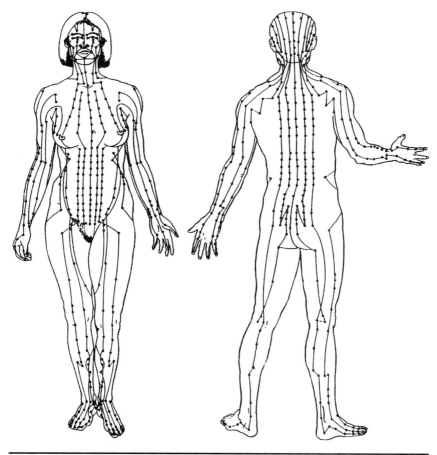

Figure 2–3. Acupuncture points.
Source. From *Between Heaven and Earth* by Harriet Beinfield and Efram Korngold. Copyright © 1991 by Harriet Beinfield and Efram Korngold. Reprinted by permission of Ballantine Books, a division of Random House, Inc.

ment of one often stimulates the development of the others. The factors that precipitate these disease processes may attack from outside the body, arise from inside the body, or belong to a category considered neither external nor internal. Excesses mentioned above may either attack from outside or arise internally. The neither/nor factors include diet, physical activity, sexual activity, burns, bites, parasites, and trauma.

Role of Emotions

The internal factors that may precipitate disease are the emotions. The *Nei Jing,* one of the earliest texts of TCM, lists seven emotions that commonly precipitate disease if they become either excessive or deficient: Joy, Anger, Sadness, Grief, Worry and Brooding, Fear, and Fright.[1] For example, excess Joy manifests as Craving. The meaning of Craving in TCM is far broader than our association of it with addiction. Showing the influence of Taoist and Buddhist thought, Craving is considered the attempt to hold on to what is impermanent, and everything in life is considered impermanent. In this system, jealousy is a form of craving, or excess Joy.

The inseparability of mind and body is profoundly captured in the TCM understanding of emotion. Each emotion is considered to be one of the functional expressions of an Organ (see Maciocia 1994, pp. 200–217): Joy is a functional expression of the Heart, anger is an expression of the Liver, Sadness and Grief are expressions of the Lungs, Worry and Brooding are expressions of the Spleen, and Fear and Fright are expressions of the Kidneys. As functions of the Organs, emotions are healthy when they are in balance with the system as a whole and harmful when they are not. Very little attention is given to healthy emotions, but their effects can be extrapolated from the other functions of the Organs with which they are associated. Anger, for example, has the quality of a powerful, intense focus, which can direct a person toward a desired goal.

When an emotion is excessive, either because it is too intense or because it is prolonged beyond the appropriate time to focus on its object, it acts like every other precipitating factor of disease; it disrupts the Vital Substances and Organs. In particular, emotions affect the Qi and Blood. They may lead to deficiency or stagnation of Qi or to deficiency, Heat, or stagnation of Blood. When the Qi is deficient, the Spleen, Lungs, and/or Kidneys may not transform fluids, which may instead accumulate as Phlegm. When

---

[1] The exact number of emotions that may precipitate disease is subject to controversy: in some schools of thought, Sadness and Grief are considered one emotion, as are Fear and Fright. Categorization aside, there is broad agreement about their role in disease.

the Qi is stagnant, one possible effect is stagnation of Blood. Whether Blood is deficient, contains Heat, or is stagnant, one possible effect is Phlegm-Fire (Maciocia 1994, p. 226). These effects have been noted since the earliest texts in TCM. *The Inner Canon*, for example, says that "[i]n a patient full of grief and sadness, the Qi becomes depressed and does not move" (Guo Xiechun 1989, cited in H. Fruehauf, "Treatment of Mental Disorders," unpublished manuscript, 1994, p. 3). This passage from *The Inner Canon* also illustrates TCM's understanding of depression as a lessening and restraining, whether of physical or emotional functions. A fifteenth-century physician went so far as to say that "[i]f Qi and Blood exist in abundance and harmony, a person will not get sick. Once there is depression, all kinds of diseases will start to evolve. Therefore all of the body's diseases are caused by depression" (quoted in Zhang Bosou 1991; cited in H. Fruehauf, "Treatment of Mental Disorders," unpublished manuscript, 1994, p. 3).

The effects of the emotions on the Organs also follow patterns. As we have seen, each emotion has a special relationship to a particular Organ, because the nature of the emotion matches the functions of the Organ. Anger, for example, is said to injure the Liver. Remember that one of the main functions of the Liver is to ensure that Qi flows smoothly in the proper direction. The sudden, flaring nature of acute anger, which rushes toward its object, mirrors the function of directing the flow of Qi. One effect of unhealthy anger is that Qi ascends when it should descend. This may result in flushing, headache, or labile mood. The knotted, dense nature of chronic anger might result in stagnation of Qi, which may be manifested as depressed mood or flank and chest pain. In TCM, treating the mood and the pain independently is senseless at best.

The effects of the emotions on the Shen are equally important to their effects on Qi. Because Shen is a refined form of Qi, it exists everywhere that Qi exists. Each Yin Organ is said to have a Shen, and the term refers to a particular dimension of the Heart, as well as the collectivity of these dimensions of the five Yin Organs as a group (Maciocia 1994, pp. 200–217). The "Five Shen" and their organs are as follows: Shen—Heart; Ethereal Soul (*Hun*)—Liver; Corporeal Soul (*Po*)—Lungs; Intellect (*Yi*)—Spleen; and Will (*Zhi*)—Kidneys. Any and all emotional stress, regardless of origin, is capable of disrupting the flow of Qi and thereby damaging the Shen in the collective sense.

The Shen that resides in the Heart is responsible for all mental activity as well as the five senses. All perceptions and emotions are said to be recognized and felt in the Heart. In turn, anything that damages the Heart will also damage its Shen. Thus, the connection between depression and heart disease and the need to treat both simultaneously have been part of TCM for centuries. (Heart) Shen is closely related to consciousness. Loss of consciousness, lack of clarity in thought, diminished insight, and poor judgment all reflect a disturbance of the Shen.

The Ethereal Soul (*Hun*) is said to enter the body shortly after birth and survive the body after death, though not in a personalized form. It can be understood in Buddhist terms as the part of individual consciousness (Small Mind) that exemplifies universal consciousness (Big Mind). The Ethereal Soul makes its home in the Liver. If the Liver Yin and/or Blood are depleted, the Ethereal Soul loses it home and wanders. This may be expressed as insomnia, timidity, fear, or a lack or direction. Like the Shen, the Ethereal Soul participates in all mental activities. In one text it is described as the "coming and going" of the (Heart) Shen, meaning that by means of the Ethereal Soul the (Heart) Shen both manifests itself in the outside world and connects with the inner world of intuition, dreams, and the unconscious. Also, the (Heart) Shen is said to "gather" the Ethereal Soul. If the two are balanced, the person has calm wisdom. A person who has many dreams but never accomplishes anything may lack a Shen strong enough to restrain the Ethereal Soul. Within TCM, this problem cannot be described as functional or organic, as emotional or physical. The Ethereal Soul and the Shen, in this case our dreams and their expression, involve body, mind, and spirit. Disturbances of the Ethereal Soul manifest as problems of the Liver and are treated by treating that Organ and its connections. As it says in the *Spiritual Axis*, "If the liver is deficient there will be fear; if it is in excess there will be anger" (Ling Shu Jing c. 100 BC/1981, cited in Maciocia 1994, p. 203).

The Corporeal Soul (*Po*) arises soon after a person is conceived and dies with the body. Just as the Ethereal Soul is the coming and going of the (Heart) Shen and provides its movement, the Corporeal Soul is the "exiting and entering of Jing"; it provides the body the capacity for movement and allows the Jing to interact with the other Vital Substances. Corporeal Soul is also what allows us to register and feel sensations and to express them physically. Thus, it is related to the sense organs, including the skin, and plays a role in crying and weeping. It is said to "root" the Ethereal Soul, which is related to maintaining the flow of Vital Substances in the proper direction. Because the Corporeal Soul resides in the Lungs, it is closely associated with breathing. Thus, in meditation, breathing is used to quiet the Corporeal Soul, which roots the Ethereal Soul and thereby calms mental activity, strengthens the Shen, and increases insight. Emotional tensions that express themselves as pain, skin rashes, and/or itching are described as disturbances of the Corporeal Soul. *Yi* has been translated both as intellect and as intention. Among other things it is responsible for the application of mental activity to specific tasks (e.g., memorizing information for use in study or work). The lack of concentration common in depression may be related to a disturbance of Yi, or the Spleen, where it resides. Unchecked, the Yi can lead to melancholic brooding or obsessive compulsion. *Zhi*, like the Shen, has multiple meanings (Bensky 1992). The one most relevant for us is purpose, will, or ambition. It is a person's sense of what to focus on, where to put one's efforts, and what one ultimately wants to be. A lack of Will may be an important part of depression. The Will is associated with the Kidney, which stores the Jing. Just as Jing provides a kind of physical substrate for the Shen, Will is essential for achieving the desires of the (Heart) Shen.

Traditional Chinese Medicine in Practice

If TCM were only a sophisticated and elegant theory of the human terrain of health and disease, it would not have survived in contemporary medicine. And if Qi and Shen were merely metaphors, no techniques for assessing them would have interobserver reliability. Such is not the case. In addition to taking a detailed history, the two major ways that a person's health is assessed by a TCM practitioner are examination of the tongue and palpation of the pulse.

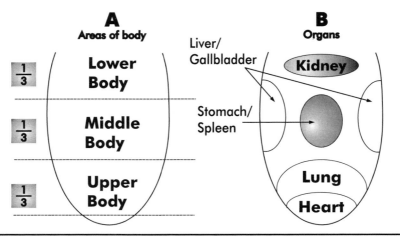

A
Areas of body

B
Organs

$\frac{1}{3}$ Lower Body

$\frac{1}{3}$ Middle Body

$\frac{1}{3}$ Upper Body

Liver/Gallbladder

Stomach/Spleen

Kidney

Lung

Heart

Figure 2–4. Relationship between areas of tongue and areas of body (**A**) and the Organs (**B**).

Tongue diagnosis (see, e.g., Maciocia 1987) has several advantages as a diagnostic technique. The condition of the tongue reflects the long-term condition of the patient and is relatively unaffected by immediate or short-term changes, such as anxiety over being examined by a doctor or running to be on time for the appointment. Changes in the tongue provide a convenient and reliable way to track whether the patient's condition is responding to treatment. There is general agreement about the correspondence between areas of the tongue and Organs (Figure 2–4) and good interobserver reliability (e.g., a pale tongue is perceived as pale, a red tongue as red). Detailed discussion here is not necessary; the point is that a TCM practitioner carefully observes the tongue and gauges the efficacy of treatment over time by whether the body, coating, and moisture of the tongue become more normal (Table 2–2).

Pulse diagnosis is an extraordinarily complex topic. What is important for our purposes is that the TCM practitioner palpates the pulse at three positions on each wrist. In some systems, each position is palpated at three depths: superficial, middle, and deep. Each position corresponds to a different area of the body and to different Organs. The pulse is palpated not just for rate and rhythm but also for 28 separate qualities. Depending on the quality of the pulse and the location in which that quality is palpated, a diag-

Table 2–2. Tongue diagnosis

Tongue	Aspect	Clinical significance
Vitality of color		Overall prognosis
Body	Color	Qi, Blood, Yin Organs
	Shape	Qi, Blood, Yin Organs
Coating	Color	Hot/Cold
	Thickness	Strength of Pernicious Influence/ strength of Qi
	Distribution	Progression of External Pernicious Influence/location of Internal Pernicious Influence
	Root	Strength of Qi, especially Kidney and Stomach
Moisture		Depletion/accumulation of bodily fluids

nosis is hypothesized. Although complex and difficult to learn, pulse diagnosis is the most impressive diagnostic technique developed in TCM. Experienced practitioners are able to "read" the pulse and give a detailed history of the patient's condition, list the patient's symptoms, and pinpoint the location of the disharmony even without knowing anything about the patient. To the uninformed it looks like wizardry. The limitation of both pulse and tongue diagnosis in modern medicine is the ability of some medications to alter the quality of the pulse and the condition of the tongue. Some of these effects are predictable and can be factored out, whereas others are just being discovered and their interference with diagnostic accuracy is unknown.

Let's take the example of a person who complains of depressed mood to illustrate how the process of diagnosis proceeds (Figure 2–5). The term *yuzheng* (depression syndrome) encompasses numerous symptoms that are usually precipitated by emotions (see central box in Figure 2–5). It may also be precipitated by poor diet (which weakens the Spleen); overwork (which includes what we call exercise and may deplete Vital Substances, including Kidney Jing); medications, illicit drugs, or alcohol (which may injure the Liver or, in severe cases, the Kidney); or blood loss or any prolonged illness (which may lead to deficiency of any Vital Substance

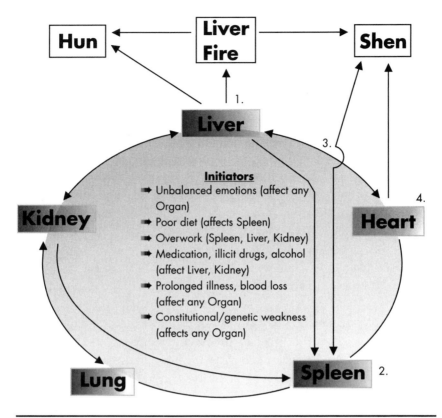

Figure 2–5. Pathophysiology of depression in traditional Chinese medicine. The major relationships among Organs in the pathogenesis of depression are depicted. Examples are 1) Stagnant Liver Qi generates Fire and affects the Spleen; 2) Deficient Spleen Qi results in accumulation of Phlegm, which affects the Heart; 3) Deficiency in Liver and Heart disturb the Hun and Shen; and 4) Deficiency in Heart disturbs the Shen.

or Organ). All emotions, as we know, may injure the Heart. But in general, acute emotions affect the Qi, particularly of the Liver. Their most common acute effect is Liver Qi stagnation. Over time, emotions may result in severe stagnation, which may generate Fire; deficiency, which may drain Vital Substances from a variety of Organs; or failure to transform, with subsequent accumulation of excess Phlegm or Damp.

Whereas in Western medicine the analytic process is differential diagnosis, in which either/or choices are repeatedly made until ideally a single entity is selected as the cause, in TCM the practitioner discerns patterns of symptoms, pulse, and tongue to choose a point of intervention. For example, someone complaining of depressed mood, restlessness, poor appetite, blurry vision, and nausea who has a "wiry" pulse exhibits a pattern of Stagnant Liver Qi, with Liver Affecting the Spleen (numeral 1 in Figure 2–5). In Five Phases theory, this is an example of Wood (the Liver) controlling Earth (the Spleen). Acupoints would be selected to restore the flow of Qi in the Liver and to build the Spleen. If, however, the patient complained of a feeling of something's being stuck in the throat, some swelling in the limbs, bloating after eating, and stuffiness in the chest (numeral 2 in Figure 2–5), and he or she had a "slippery" pulse and a sticky tongue coating, points would be added to resolve Phlegm, and perhaps to build the Spleen Qi. A depressed patient complaining of dizziness, excessive dreaming at night, timidity, insomnia, and forgetfulness (numeral 3 in Figure 2–5) with a pale tongue and a thin pulse is exhibiting a pattern of Deficient Liver and Heart Blood, disturbed Hun, and a disturbed Shen. In Five Phases theory, Wood is not producing Fire. Points would be chosen to calm the Shen, root the Hun, and build the Liver and Heart Blood. To give just one more example, a patient with uncontrollable crying, inability to concentrate, restless sleep, and a feeling of being out of control (numeral 4 in Figure 2–5) who has a midline crack in the body of the tongue and a red tip accompanied by a hollow and rapid pulse has a disharmony primarily involving the Heart. Points to quiet and build the Shen and build Yin would be chosen. At subsequent visits it is likely that at least some points would change as the pattern of symptoms, pulse, and tongue responded to the treatment. Although some standardization exists and some points are particularly useful for specific symptoms, the individuation of treatments based on close observation remains the heart of TCM.

Acupuncture and Biomedical Research

Just as every person speaks with an accent, usually inaudible to the speaker, every medical system and scientific practice is shaped by the culture in which it develops and is used. When an economically and politically dominant country or group of countries develops a particular practice, it generally becomes exported/imposed on the rest of the world. It would be odd if contemporary psychiatry followed a different course. Medicine has not entered the postmodernist age; the culture of medicine presupposes that there is one reality, discoverable by an unambiguous experimental method. The "hard" science of medicine is biologically based, and psychiatry simply awaits the discovery of the biochemical markers that will allow it to isolate, analyze, and develop cures for all mental illnesses.

This conception of psychiatry is akin to the search for pathogens during the development of infectious disease as a specialty. Find the bug, develop the drug, and you've done your job and done humanity a service. This attitude prompted much valuable research, but it is now well recognized that public health measures focusing on environmental strategies for control of infectious agents are the main reason for the dramatic decline in infectious disease that accompanied the development of antibiotics. Antibiotics are unquestionably useful, life-saving, and important, but preventive measures affect more people, have far more social benefits, and produce no side effects. At least some psychiatrists believe, similarly, that although the discovery of biochemical markers of mental disorders is an aid, we cannot assume that these markers will provide all, or even the most important, answers to the question of how best to treat mental disorders. Some support for this view is found in the experiences of other cultures.

Psychiatry and Culture

In psychiatry the challenge to biological reductionism is to explain the interactions among history, culture, and mental disorders. At least three kinds of questions force attention to these issues. First, if mental disease is primarily biological, why are some mental disorders culture-specific? The appendix to DSM-IV (American Psychiatric Association 1994) lists *amok* and *latah* as culture-specific but does not recognize anorexia nervosa, multiple personality disorder, or chronic fatigue syndrome as culture-bound (Kleinman and Cohen 1997). For that matter, in traditional cultures an excess of any emotion is considered harmful, but modern psychiatry focuses on just three: excess sadness is termed *depression*, excess fear is termed *anxiety* (Wig 1990), and excess happiness is termed *mania*. That excess anger is not in itself considered pathologic seems more a reflection of the cultures in which modern psychiatry developed than a reflection of what creates suffering in people's lives. Second, if mental disease is primarily biological, why are there different prevalence rates in different parts of the world, and among different socioeconomic classes? Even schizophrenia, which is the strongest candidate for a biologically based mental disease, varies in prevalence in different parts of the world (Kleinman and Cohen 1997; Wen 1998), which at least suggests the influence of culture. Voluminous evidence exists indicating that rates of depression, anxiety, and other mental problems vary by class and degree of stigmatization. Third, historical changes result in varying rates of particular mental disorders. Should we conclude then that industrialization produces changes in biology?

In mainstream psychiatry, recognition of cultural difference is expressed in the distinction between disease and illness, with disease referring to biological processes and illness referring to the personal and cultural expression or construction of disease (e.g., Eisenbruch 1983). This is also referred to as the "pathogenicity/pathoplasticity dichotomy." In addition to the fact that varying prevalence rates challenge the assumption on which the dichotomy rests, use of a dichotomy is itself culture-bound. Preoccupation with dichotomies is a prominent feature of the European tradition in psychiatry (Wig 1990). Debates over the relative importance of nature/nurture, thinking/feeling, body/mind, conscious/unconscious, and organic/functional stem from seeing these as contrasting opposites rather than placing them in a context of juxtaposition and identification of polarities (Mora 1980) as in Yin-Yang theory.

The clearest expression of the differences between the two approaches surrounds what DSM-IV calls somatoform disorders. The implication is that the "real" cause of the patient's complaints is psychologic and that the physical symptoms are "masking" psychic conflicts and disturbances that the patient is unable to face or that are "maladaptive" ways of coping with conflict. This category cannot exist in TCM because there is no distinction between mind and body and there is no cause hiding behind the expression of disease. Rather than "excluding" an "organic" cause, TCM practitioners treat what they find, along whatever point in the biological/mental continuum. Open any standard acupuncture text and examine the lists of indications for acupoints and you will find "somatic" and "psychic" indications listed together. For example, common indications for the fifth point on the Bladder Channel are headache, blurring of vision, and epilepsy; for the seventh point on the Pericardium Channel they include cardiac pain, vomiting, palpitations, panic, mental disorders, and pain in the chest and hypochondriac region (Beijing, Shanghai, and Nanjing College of Traditional Chinese Medicine 1980). Whether a pattern is "maladaptive" or normative depends in large part on how it is perceived and handled by the community. The advantage of TCM is that it neither privileges nor denigrates either the physical or the psychologic. It reframes the patient's symptoms in a pattern encompassing both mental and physical factors. In this way it avoids the stigmatization of mental illness while highlighting the patterns existing in and partly created by the person. The metaphoric nature of the language of TCM works to its advantage here. Tell a depressed person that he or she is "stuck" or needs to "nourish" a deficiency, and if your diagnosis is right, the words resonate with the person's experience and offer an opening for a dialogue about behavioral changes.

Research on Acupuncture

Contemporary scientific investigations into the efficacy of acupuncture have almost all been conducted within a biological reductionist model. Perhaps because widespread attention to acupuncture in the biomedical community followed President Nixon's trip to China, during which James Reston had an emergency appendectomy under acupuncture analgesia, early research focused on acupuncture for pain control, and subsequent research has focused primarily on acupuncture's effect on the nervous system. Explaining all the effects of acupuncture in terms of culturally acceptable concepts such as neurotransmitters would obviate the need to refer to concepts like Qi, which many regard as disreputably metaphysical. For example, "de Qi," a sensation of heaviness, numbness, or aching at the site of needle insertion and sometimes radiating from there has been hypothesized to result from the activation of type II and III muscle sensory nerves (Pomeranz 1996). Andersson and Lundeberg (1995) asserted that low-frequency electrical stimulation, such as that sometimes used on acupuncture needles, activates mechanoreceptors in multiple tissue types. They speculated that, through this mechanism, acupuncture has physiologic effects on afferent input in somatic nerve fibers similar to those of physical exercise. This hypothesis awaits further research. If true, acupuncture might, for example, have an effect on mild depression similar to that of exercise.

Although exact mechanisms are still under investigation, it is well established that acupuncture acts on the nervous system locally, regionally, and centrally. Locally, acupuncture stimulates vasoactive intestinal peptide and a host of inflammatory mediators. It is also known to affect the spinal cord, midbrain, and hypothalamus/pituitary in a way that stimulates the release of enkephalins, dynorphins, β-endorphins, calcitonin gene-related peptide, methionine, adrenocorticotropic hormone (ACTH), serotonin, norepinephrine, and dopamine (Han 1986; Pomeranz 1996; Stux and Pomeranz 1987, 1991; Tsou 1987, 1989), and to regulate the balance between the sympathetic and parasympathetic nervous systems (Andersson and Lundeberg 1995; Karavis 1997). Many of these substances are known to be important in the pathophysiology of mental diseases, and their regulation suggests that acupuncture could play a role in treating mental illness. In light of this evidence, even those averse to notions such as Qi and Shen could reasonably ask whether acupuncture would benefit depression, anxiety, or schizophrenia.

A review of the literature disappoints anyone looking for conclusive evidence (Table 2–3). Most studies on the use of acupuncture for mental disorders are case series. Blinding is rare. Randomized trials, when they exist, are of very low quality: enrollment procedures, eligibility criteria, definitions of treatment, length of treatment, and number of acupuncture sessions are often unspecified. When specified, they vary tremendously from one study to the next, which makes it difficult to sum the effects of multiple small studies. In short, there is insufficient evidence to make recommendations about acupuncture for the treatment of mental disorders on the basis of existing trials. Except for the issue of addiction, for which it found insufficient evidence, the National Institutes of Health (NIH) Consensus Statement on Acupuncture (1997) does not even address mental disorders. Two conclusions can be drawn from these facts. First, what acupuncturists do in practice is not based on clinical trials. Second, the methodologic infrastructure for assessing acupuncture does not yet exist (Margolin et al. 1998).

Although the evidence that acupuncture is effective for treating mental disorders is inconclusive, there are several reasons to continue to study it. Eight of the trials cited above directly compared acupuncture with standard treatment and found no statistical difference between the two. The NIH Consensus Statement (1997) found evidence suggesting that acupuncture was effective in the treatment of conditions such as postoperative pain and postchemotherapy nausea and that acupuncture is effective in numerous other conditions, including asthma, dysmenorrhea, and osteoarthritis. The variety of mechanisms that produce these conditions and the contribution of anxiety to some of them suggest that we are far from understanding the true scope of acupuncture's effects. In addition, people in every class and from a multitude of cultures use acupuncture as their treatment of choice (Eisenberg et al. 1993). Although continuance of a procedure over time is not in itself evidence for its effectiveness, its continuity over time and across cultures, coupled with widespread contemporary use, demands the attention of serious physicians.

Two other conclusions can be drawn from any general survey of acupuncture research for any problem (see, e.g., Helms 1995, pp. 42–56). First, acupuncture is safe. After literally millions of treatments, only five fatalities were reported in the literature from 1965 through 1996 (Ernst and White 1997). The greatest risks are infection, which results from improper use or reuse of needles without sterilization, and pneumothorax. The use of disposable needles, which is nearly universal in the United States and Japan,

Table 2–3. Trials of acupuncture for mental disorders

Study	Clinical problem	N	Type of trial	Treatment	Quality	Outcome
Kane and DiScipio 1979	Schizophrenia	3	Case report	BA vs. sham acupuncture	Low	2 of 3 responded positively to BA but not to sham acupuncture
Shi and Tan 1986	Schizophrenia	500	Case series	EAR and BA; some patients given chlorpromazine	Low	55% cured; 16.8% greatly improved
Zheng and Xiu 1988	Psychotic hallucinations	216	Case series	EAR vs. EAR, BA vs. EAR, and 200 mg chlorpromazine	Low	No statistically significant differences among groups
Zhang 1988	Hallucinations	296	Case series	BA	Low	70.6% cured; 18.9% greatly improved
Wu 1995	Schizophrenia	53	Case series	BA, herbs	Low	100% cured
Jia et al. 1987	Schizophrenia	37	Case series	Laser acupuncture vs. 250–500 mg chlorpromazine	Low	No statistically significant differences between groups; no side effects in acupuncture group

Table 2–3. Trials of acupuncture for mental disorders (*continued*)

Study	Clinical problem	N	Type of trial	Treatment	Quality	Outcome
Zhang 1987	Schizophrenia	182	Randomized, unblinded trial	EA and herbs vs. EA vs. herbs vs. chlorpromazine	Low	Significantly less effect with herbs alone; no statistically significant differences among other groups
Zhou et al. 1997	Schizophrenia	40	Randomized, single-blind trial	Neuroleptics vs. EA and 40% of previous daily dose of neuroleptic	Low	No statistically significant differences between groups; fewer side effects in EA group
Zhang et al. 1987	Hysterical paralysis	1,316	Case series	BA	Low	97.8% cured
Luo et al. 1985	Depression	47	Randomized, unblinded trial	EA vs. amitriptyline	Low	No statistically significant differences among groups; fewer side effects in EA group
Luo et al. 1998	Depression	Phase I: 29	Randomized clinical trial	EA vs. amitriptyline vs. EA and amitriptyline	Low	No significant differences among groups
		Phase II: 241		EA vs. amitriptyline	Low	Significantly fewer side effects in EA group

Table 2–3. Trials of acupuncture for mental disorders *(continued)*

Study	Clinical problem	N	Type of trial	Treatment	Quality	Outcome
Allen et al. 1998	Depression	38	Randomized clinical trial crossover	BA for depression vs. BA for other symptoms vs. wait-list	Adequate	BA for depression showed statistically significant differences from BA for other symptoms; no statistically significant differences from wait-list, but in crossover, wait-list showed significant differences after BA compared with before
Liu 1998	Anxiety	240	Randomized clinical trial	EAR and BA vs. behavior therapy vs. combined	Low	No statistically significant differences between EAR and BA vs. behavior therapy; combined group two times better than other groups
Lewis 1987	Preoperation anxiety	90	Randomized clinical trial	Diazepam vs. no-needle EAR vs. relaxation tape	Adequate	No statistically significant differences in effectiveness among groups

Note. BA = body acupuncture; EA = electroacupuncture; EAR = ear acupuncture.

minimizes or eliminates the risk of infection. Sixty-five cases of pneumothorax have been reported worldwide (Ernst and White 1997). Care in needling particular points on the thorax minimizes, but does not eliminate, this risk. Overall, then, the risk is extremely low. Second, most people experience a deep sense of relaxation during acupuncture treatments. This experience is so common that trials to assess the efficacy of acupuncture for anxiety (Lewis 1987) and for prevention of opiate and other drug withdrawal (Margolin et al. 1998) often choose relaxation training as a control for acupuncture treatment. Take a theory that nonjudgmentally stresses the connections among different aspects of the person and between actions and their consequences. Couple it with a practice that is nonverbal (and, therefore, independent of education, literacy, articulateness, or insight), is relaxing, and provides a degree of personal attention and interaction; make it comparatively free of side effects and complications; and if effective, such a modality has the potential to provide relief for many patients currently considered difficult to treat by standard biomedical practice.

Methodologic Problems

Randomized controlled trials constitute one appropriate design to test the efficacy of drugs. But acupuncture is not a drug. It is a procedure (diagnosis, selection of treatment, and treatment) that relies on a device (the needle and its accessories) to deliver its effects. By now there is near-universal agreement that trials of acupuncture cannot be double-blind. Using people untrained in acupuncture to insert needles cannot guarantee a minimum standard of care (Hammerschlag 1998; Lewith and Machin 1983; Vincent and Richardson 1986). Single-blind studies are not impossible to design, as will be seen below, but problems other than blinding are more difficult to solve.

The barriers to specifying the model for testing acupuncture can be grouped into two main categories: 1) developing treatment protocols and 2) selecting appropriate controls and control conditions. The extent of the difficulties is apparent from the literature on ear acupuncture for addiction. Ear acupuncture itself is a non-traditional form first developed by the French physician Paul Nogier in the 1940s. Ear acupuncture as a method of treating the craving for substances began in the 1970s. Dr. Wen, a neurosurgeon in Hong Kong, was researching acupuncture analgesia. When several of his opiate-addicted trial participants reported decreased withdrawal symptoms, he began to study acupuncture as a treatment for opiate addiction. No complex theoretical underpinnings trouble this technique, which is a purely empirically based invention. Symptoms determine point selection, and the treatment protocol is not controversial. Still, variations in selection of appropriate controls and methods to eliminate bias have rendered the literature on the use of acupuncture for addiction inconclusive. The best-designed trial, the Cocaine Alternative Treatments Study, is under way as of this writing (Margolin et al. 1998) and will be an important step in the development of acupuncture research. The barriers to adequate research on the use of acupuncture in the treatment of other mental disorders are even more formidable.

Treatment Protocols

For treatment of mental disorders, unlike that of addiction, the TCM diagnostic category potentially affects point selection. As was noted earlier, two people diagnosed with depression by DSM-IV criteria might well be given two different diagnoses by TCM practitioners. In addition, although the diagnosis does not change during the treatment process in Western psychiatry unless it is believed that an error was made, in TCM it is expected that the pattern of dysfunction will change in response to treatment and that the treatment will change accordingly. Some acupuncturists have nonetheless developed a "cookbook" approach in which the same set of points is needled in everyone with a particular symptom or with a particular Western disease diagnosis. This approach is more warranted the narrower the condition being addressed. For example, needling Pericardium 6 has been investigated in the treatment of nausea, whether it be from pregnancy, chemotherapy, seasickness, weakness of Stomach or Spleen Qi, invasion of the Spleen by the Liver, or retention of food. But the clinical manifestations of depression are far more complex and varied than nausea.

We have seen that acupuncture points are selected according to clinical manifestations. In clinical practice point selection is adjusted not just individual by individual but also by symptom complex (pattern) presentation at each visit. Furthermore, treatment of the whole person by expelling excesses, strengthening, or balancing is a vital element of the overall treatment plan and will differ from individual to individual. Using the same set of points for everyone with the same Western diagnosis of a mental disorder is as senseless as predetermining the issues that can be discussed with patients by psychotherapists in order to test different theories of anxiety, or prescribing penicillin to everyone with a fever in order to "test antibiotics." No adequate trial of acupuncture for mental disorders can avoid incorporating variation in TCM diagnosis and in subsequent point selection.

Assuming we have solved the problem of selecting points, we have a variety of methods available for stimulating those points. We could needle them, stimulate them with electricity with or without needling them, tape small pellets with or without magnets onto the points and instruct people to manually stimulate the pellets as symptoms arise, or burn small cones of the herb *Artemisia vulgaris* (moxa) either directly onto the point or onto a needle inserted into the point. All of these procedures are routinely employed in clinical practice. Without trials it is premature to assume that one method is superior to another. Some pain studies suggest that analgesic effect is enhanced by electricity, but these studies have compared electric stimulation only with needles without electricity. No trials have compared electroacupuncture with manual stimulation of needles or with needles with moxa. Developing treatment protocols is impossible without resolving these questions.

Once points are selected and the stimulation method is decided, the correct "dose" of acupuncture has to be determined. Dose includes intensity of stimulation, duration of needle retention, and number of total treatments. Having discovered that many acupuncture points overlap with trigger points (Melzack et al. 1977) and motor points (Liu et al. 1977), researchers seemed to conclude that the Western mechanism explained the effect of acupuncture points and that depth of insertion determined outcome. This mirrors the assumption of most Chinese acupuncturists that unless "de Qi" is felt, the treatment will not be effective and that when treating pain, the stronger the sensations felt from the needles the more effective the treatment will be.[2] However, other acupuncturists in the Chinese and other traditions, notably in Japan, do not believe "de Qi" is necessary for an effective treatment and do not routinely elicit it, or they believe it is only necessary for certain conditions or individuals. Are these cultural differences? Does acupuncture work by many, currently unknown mechanisms? What depth is appropriate for what points in which clinical situations? Is intense stimulation more appropriate for some disorders than others? Does intensity of stimulation influence the number of total treatments necessary for a cure? Does this differ from disorder to disorder? From individual to individual? Without knowing the answers to these questions, how can we say that a particular treatment has failed?

Controls in Acupuncture Research

The two most difficult problems in eliminating bias from acupuncture research are how to control for participant bias and how to select an appropriate control treatment. Participant bias arises because of interactions between the patients and the practitioners or because of the beliefs of the patient. Margolin et al. (1998) have limited verbal exchanges between patient and practitioner by allowing practitioners to answer questions without elaboration but proscribing them from initiating exchanges or conversation and by having a third person monitor all interactions. This innovation provides additional rigor to their study. It does not, however, control for nonverbal interactions between patient and practitioner.

The Qi in the body is not considered separate from the Qi in the universe. Exchanges of Qi between people are considered not just possible but commonplace. Indeed, the whole discipline of Qi

---

[2] What many Chinese persons perceive as a good, strong, satisfying treatment, most Americans perceive as unacceptably painful. This cultural difference has led to a situation in which some standard treatments in China are rarely if ever done in the United States.

Gong is a highly developed system for training people to build their own and others' Qi and to transfer Qi from one person to another. What Westerners call "charisma" and "star power" is considered a teachable skill within TCM, although both traditions recognize that some people, trained or not, seem to have more of it than others. How do we control for practitioners who have acupuncture star power—the nonverbal ability to direct and build the flow of Qi in their patients? Should we control for it, or should we be training all practitioners to develop it as best they can? There are many types of star power, and there are many configurations of Qi. Some people think Tom Cruise looks boring, and some people's Qi matches with a given individual better than others. If these may be confounding factors, we need to develop controls for them.

Other nonverbal exchanges may also influence outcomes. Consider the attitude of the practitioner. Suppose having an attitude of unconditional love for the patient influences outcomes. (This is a belief very widely held among practitioners of complementary and alternative medicine.) Can we assume that unconditional love does not affect outcome? How do we limit this sort of exchange? There are some parallels between these questions and questions raised about psychotherapy. Is the person more important than the psychotherapeutic theory? In comparing psychotherapies, is the relationship with the patient, the "fit" between patient and practitioner, more important than the method?

We could push these questions even further and ask about the "fit" between the patient and the environment. Just as some people have more Qi than others, some places and arrangements of the environment are considered to have more Qi than others. Does this mean that certain places in the world, where there is an abundance of Qi, are more "healing," or that certain environments are more healing? Given that Qi circulates and accumulates in the body in cycles, are there times of day for which certain conditions should be treated? seasons of the year? Could all of these be confounding factors in studies, or should they be considered part of a "good" treatment?

By comparison with controlling interactions with patients, controlling for patient belief in the procedure or confidence in the practitioner is more easily accomplished. The Treatment Credibility Scale (Borkevic and Nau 1972), which evaluates the relative credibility of different psychotherapies, has been adapted for acupuncture research (Vincent 1990). The Working Alliance Inventory, which evaluates the bond between patient and practitioner and their agreement on goals and tasks, has been modified by Margolin et al. (1998) for use in acupuncture research. But what about other patient factors? Perhaps certain constitutions or genetic endowments are more suitable for acupuncture and should be controlled for. Shared beliefs are as important as individual beliefs. What if there is something about the needling process, within certain cultures or subgroups of individuals, that makes the acupuncture session a particularly apt healing ritual? How do we discover that?

Finally, having settled these issues, we have to choose an appropriate control for acupuncture treatment (Vincent and Lewith 1995). Hammerschlag (1998) discusses five categories of controls: wait-list, placebo, sham, comparison with biomedical standard care, and adjunctive to biomedical standard care. In this classification, the difference between placebo and sham is that placebo controls are noninvasive (e.g., mock needling or mock transcutaneous electrical nerve stimulation [TENS]). Many studies have used so-called sham points, which are not located on Channels but are close to recognized acupoints, to serve as controls. Because we have no Western definition of what constitutes an acupuncture point, how do we know what is a "sham" point? The NIH Consensus Panel (1997, p. 8) noted that, especially in pain studies, sham acupuncture often has effects either intermediate between "placebo" and "real" acupuncture or effects similar to "real" acupuncture. Within TCM there is the tradition of needling so-called *Ah Shi* points. They are located by palpation, usually tender, and not necessarily on any of the Channels. How do we know whether a point is sham or Ah Shi? Furthermore, because Qi is conceived of as being present everywhere in the body, it is theoretically possible that any point has some effect. No consensus yet exists about how to resolve this problem.

If we conceive of the effects of acupuncture as due to placebo, nonspecific physiologic responses to skin piercing, and specific responses to stimulation of particular points (Hammerschlag 1998), then the advantage of sham acupuncture is that it works well as a control for the first two. The disadvantage is that a much larger number of subjects may be required for a study to have the power to detect treatment differences (Vincent and Richardson 1986). Thompson (1980) noted that when comparing tricyclic antidepressants with an active placebo (which produced a dry mouth), only one in seven trials showed a superior effect for the drug. In contrast, Morris and Beck (1974) found that 65% of double-blind trials showed tricyclics to be superior to inert placebos. Also, as Hammerschlag (1998) points out, both placebo and sham acupuncture raise bioethical concerns by violating the "intent to treat" principle. One way to avoid this problem when treating chronic conditions is to provide acupuncture to control group patients at the end of the trial (Jobst et al. 1986). For more acute conditions, acupuncture versus standard biomedical care or standard biomedical care with acupuncture versus standard biomedical care without acupuncture are the ethical treatment designs.

In summary, the methodologic shortcomings of research on acupuncture all stem from a common source: we have not asked whether acupuncture is an effective TCM treatment, we have asked whether acupuncture needles can be used within Western biomedical diagnosis and treatment (see, e.g., Hammerschlag 1998; Hammerschlag and Morris 1997). This approach may have some merit in other areas, but in psychiatry it is unjustifiable. To begin with, it is inherently illogical. Because we do not have sufficient biomedical markers for mental disorders and do not completely understand the physiologic mechanisms by which they occur, we have no definitive way to test acupuncture as a biomedical treatment. Furthermore, by ignoring TCM diagnosis when selecting points for treating patients, trials of acupuncture have introduced a bias that diminishes the potential power of the treatment.

Future Directions

A new generation of clinical trials is needed in which TCM and biomedical models are directly compared. In such trials, people with a particular biomedical diagnosis also would be diagnosed within TCM. Point selection in the acupuncture group would vary by TCM diagnosis and could vary from treatment to treatment, as long as appropriate clinical manifestations were cited to justify the change (e.g., added Stomach 40 because patient developed nausea, thick white tongue coat, and slippery pulse, indicating Dampness). Patients in the nonacupuncture group also would be diagnosed according to TCM, and subgroup analysis would compare TCM categories in the two groups. Then we could begin to learn which people respond better to which model.

However, this leads us to a final complication. Acupuncture is only a small part of TCM. Of the three types of disease processes, acupuncture is most effective when there is stagnation or obstruction, relatively effective when there is accumulation of excess due to failure to transform, and least effective when a person's primary problem is deficiency. Herbs may be appropriate for any disease process, but in the last two cases most practitioners will almost always prescribe herbs in addition to acupuncture. We are nowhere near being able to design trials, let alone conduct them, to determine whether acupuncture, acupuncture plus herbs, herbs alone, or standard biomedical treatment is optimal for a given individual. But even in mainstream medicine this is the face of the future. The guidelines published in the Joint National Committee's report on high blood pressure (1997) are a good example of this direction. Choice of initial antihypertensive now depends on comorbidities. This recognition, that the condition (the strength) of the individual and the entire constellation of problems he or she manifests must be taken into account before deciding on treatment, is a fundamental principle of TCM.

Wig (1990) pointed out that no single medical system has ever been the sole method by which people seek healing. Parallel systems with differing and often incompatible principles and varying degrees of evidential support are the norm throughout human history, not the exception. Acupuncture is safe and relaxing. It has known physiologic effects that suggest its usefulness for a wide variety of conditions. It also provides both a theory and practice of harmony and balance within and among individuals, communities, and the environment that encourage critical reflection on the biomedical standard of care.

The sophisticated phenomenologic descriptions of health and disease in TCM offer an approach to conditions such as somatization that may be particularly appealing to patients. Adequate research on the application of acupuncture and other modalities within TCM to the treatment of mental disorders will stimulate the development of all approaches to these problems.

Perhaps the greatest value of TCM, whether it is used as a first choice, an alternative, or an adjunct to biomedical care, is its emphasis not on treating mental illness but on restoring mental health. It conceptualizes the individual in a nexus of community and nature, but it always places the individual at the center of treatment.

References

Acupuncture. NIH Consensus Statement. 15(5):1–34, November 3–5, 1997

Allen J, Schnyer R, Hitt S: The efficacy of acupuncture in the treatment of major depression in women. Psychological Sciences 9:397–401, 1998

American Psychiatric Association: Diagnostic and Statistical Manual of Mental Disorders, 4th Edition. Washington, DC, American Psychiatric Association, 1994

Andersson S, Lundeberg T: Acupuncture—from empiricism to science: functional background to acupuncture effects in pain and disease. Med Hypotheses 45:271–281, 1995

Beijing, Shanghai, and Nanjing Colleges of Traditional Chinese Medicine, The Acupuncture Institute of the Academy of Traditional Chinese Medicine: Essentials of Chinese Acupuncture. Beijing, Foreign Languages Press, 1980

Bensky D: Purpose, elation and the pancreas. American Association of Medical Acupuncture Review 4:24–28, 1992

Borkevic TD, Nau SD: Credibility of analogue therapy rationales. J Behav Ther Exp Psychiatry 3:257–260, 1972

Eisenberg DM, Kessler RC, Foster C, et al: Unconventional medicine in the United States: prevalence, costs, and patterns of use. N Engl J Med 328:246–252, 1993

Eisenbruch M: Wind illness or somatic depression? A case study in psychiatric anthropology. Br J Psychiatry 143:323–326, 1983

Ernst E, White A: Life-threatening reactions after acupuncture? A systematic review. Pain 71:123–126, 1997

Guo Xiechun (ed): Huangdi Neijing Lingshu Jiaozhu (Chapter 8). Tianjin, People's Republic of China, Tianjin Kexue Jishu, 1989, p 82

Hammerschlag R: Methodological and ethical issues in clinical trials of acupuncture. J Altern Complement Med 4:159–171, 1998

Hammerschlag R, Morris MM: Clinical trials comparing acupuncture with biomedical standard care: a criteria-based evaluation of research design and reporting. Complementary Therapies in Medicine 5:133–140, 1997

Han JS: Electroacupuncture: an alternative to antidepressants for treating affective diseases? Int J Neurosci 29:79–92, 1986

Helms JH: Acupuncture Energetics: A Clinical Approach for Physicians. Berkeley, CA, Medical Acupuncture Publishers, 1995

Jia Y, Luo H, Zhan L, et al: A study of the treatment of schizophrenia with He-Ne laser irradiation of acupoint. Journal of Traditional Chinese Medicine 7:269–272, 1987

Jobst K, Chen JH, McPherson K, et al: Controlled trials of acupuncture for disabling breathlessness. Lancet 2:1416–1419, 1986

Joint National Committee: The sixth report of the Joint National Committee on detection, evaluation, and treatment of high blood pressure. Arch Intern Med 157:2413–2416, 1997

Kane J, DiScipio W: Acupuncture treatment of schizophrenia: report on three cases. Am J Psychiatry 136:297–302, 1979

Kaptchuk T: The Web That Has No Weaver. New York, Congdon & Weed, 1983

Karavis M: The neurophysiology of acupuncture: a viewpoint. Acupuncture in Medicine 15:33–42, 1997

Kleinman A, Cohen A: Psychiatry's global challenge. Sci Am 276:86–89, 1997

Lewis GBH: An alternative approach to premedication: comparing diazepam with auriculotherapy and a relaxation method. Am J Acupunct 15:205–214, 1987

Lewith G, Machin D: On the evaluation of the clinical effects of acupuncture. Pain 16:111–127, 1983

Liu H: Illustrative cases treated by the application of the extra point sishencong. Journal of Traditional Chinese Medicine 18(2):111–114, 1988

Liu YK, Varela M, Oswald R: The correspondence between some motor points and acupuncture loci. Am J Chin Med 3:347–358, 1977

Luo H, Jia Y, Zhan L: Electro-acupuncture vs. amitriptyline in the treatment of depressive states. Journal of Traditional Chinese Medicine 5:3–8, 1985

Luo H, Meng F, Jia Y, et al: Clinical research on the therapeutic effect of the electro-acupuncture treatment in patients with depression. Psychiatry Clin Neurosci 52(suppl):S338–S340, 1998

Maciocia G: Tongue Diagnosis in Chinese Medicine. Seattle, WA, Eastland Press, 1987

Maciocia G: The Practice of Chinese Medicine. New York, Churchill Livingstone, 1994

Margolin A, Avants K, Kleber H: Rationale and design of the Cocaine Alternative Treatments Study (CATS): a randomized controlled trial of acupuncture. J Altern Complement Med 4:405–418, 1998

Melzack R, Stillwell DM, Fox J: Trigger points and acupuncture points for pain: correlations and implications. Pain 3:3–23, 1977

Mora G: Historical and theoretical trends in psychiatry, in Comprehensive Textbook of Psychiatry, Vol 1. Edited by Kaplan HI, Freedman AM, Sadock BJ. Baltimore, MD, Williams & Wilkins, 1980, pp 4–98

Morris J, Beck A: The efficacy of anti-depressant drugs: a review of research. Arch Gen Psychiatry 30:667–674, 1974

O'Connor J, Bensky D (eds): Acupuncture: A Comprehensive Text. Translated by O'Connor J, Bensky D. Seattle, WA, Eastland Press, 1981

Pomeranz B: Scientific research into acupuncture for the relief of pain. J Altern Complement Med 2:53–60, 1996

Shi Z, Tan M: An analysis of the therapeutic effect of acupuncture treatment in 500 cases of schizophrenia. Journal of Traditional Chinese Medicine 6(2):99–104, 1986

Spiritual Axis (c. 100 BC). Beijing, People's Health Publishing House, 1981, p 49

Stux G, Pomeranz B: Acupuncture: Textbook and Atlas. Berlin, Springer-Verlag, 1987

Stux G, Pomeranz B: Basics of Acupuncture, 2nd Edition, Revised. Berlin, Springer-Verlag, 1991

Thompson R: Side effects and placebo amplification. Br J Psychiatry 140:64–68, 1980

Tsou K: Neurochemical mechanisms of acupuncture analgesia, in Neurotransmitters and Pain: Control Pain and Headache, Vol 9. Edited by Akil H, Lewis JW. Basel, Switzerland, S Karger, 1987, pp 226–283

Tsou K: Activation of enkephalinergic system by acupuncture, in Scientific Bases of Acupuncture. Edited by Pomeranz B, Stux G. Berlin, Springer-Verlag, 1989, pp 113–118

Vincent CA: Credibility assessment in trials of acupuncture. Complement Med Res 4:8–11, 1990

Vincent CA, Lewith G: Placebo controls for acupuncture studies. J R Soc Med 88:199–202, 1995

Vincent CA, Richardson PH: The evaluation of therapeutic acupuncture: concepts and methods. Pain 24:1–13, 1986

Wen J-K: Folk Belief, Illness behavior and mental health in Taiwan. Chang Gung Medical Journal 21:1–12, 1998

Wig NN: The Third-World perspective on psychiatric diagnosis and classification, in Sources and Traditions of Classification in Psychiatry. Edited by Sartorius N, Jablensky A. Göttingen, Germany, Hogrefe & Huber, 1990, pp 181–210

Wu F: Treatment of schizophrenia with acu-moxibustion and Chinese medicine. Journal of Traditional Chinese Medicine 15:106–109, 1995

Zhang Bosou (ed): Zhongyi Neike Xue. Beijing, Renmin Weisheng, 1991, p 239

Zhang Jie Bin [Classic of Categories] (1624). Beijing, People's Health Publishing Company, 1982, p 49

Zhang L, Xu S, Tang Y, et al: Comparative study of the treatment of schizophrenia with electric acupuncture, herbal decoction, and chlorpromazine. Am J Acupunct 18:11–14, 1990

Zhang M: Treatment of 296 cases of hallucination with scalp acupuncture. Journal of Traditional Chinese Medicine 8:193–194, 1988

Zhang YL, Clinical study on TCM typing in schizophrenia. Journal of Combined TCM with Western Medicine 7(9):526–528, 1987

Zhang Z, Yan B, Wang W, et al: An observation of 1316 cases of hysterical paralysis treated by acupuncture. Journal of Traditional Chinese Medicine 7:113–115, 1987

Zhou G, Jin S, Zhang L: Comparative clinical study on the treatment of schizophrenia with electroacupuncture and reduced doses of antipsychotic drugs. Am J Acupunct 25:25–31, 1997

Chapter 3

Uses of Yoga in Psychiatry and Medicine

Ina Becker, M.D., Ph.D.

In this chapter I discuss the use of yogic techniques for health and prevention and in medicine and psychiatry in the context of a review of relevant research studies. A synopsis of essential yoga practices is listed in the section on the eight limbs of yoga. Resources for further study are listed at the end of the chapter.

The History of Yoga

The word *yoga* means "union" or "to yoke" and refers to one of India's wisdom traditions, used for millennia to study, explain, and experience the mystery of the mind and the human condition. It is not a religion but an experiential philosophy, using the symbols and metaphors of its mostly Hinduist but also Buddhist cultural context in the Indian subcontinent. Yoga appears to have existed as a series of loose ideas and practices at the time of the Rig-Veda, which dates back to at least 1900 B.C. Yoga is mentioned in several hymns of the Vedic Canon and seems to have flourished in the Indus-Sarasvati civilization, an early Indian civilization that thrived on the river of Sarasvati until that time. Yogic ideas began to be more defined in the Upanishads, the sacred texts of Hinduism. Feuerstein, one of the foremost Western researchers on yoga, dates the Yoga-Upanishads to the common era. The Bhagavad Gita, composed around 500–600 B.C., is the first genuine yoga scripture. It is a part of India's grand epic, The Mahabharata, and is a dialogue between the incarnate God Krishna and his pupil, the warrior Arjuna, on the night before the battle at the banks of the Ganges River:

The central message of Lord Krishna's Song is the balancing of conventional religious and ethical activity and otherworldly ascetic goals. . . . In order to win peace and enlightenment—so Krishna declares—one need not forsake the world or one's responsibilities, even when they oblige one to go into battle. Renunciation . . . of action is good in itself, but better still is renunciation in action. . . . Life in the world and spiritual life are not inimical to each other, they can and should be cultivated simultaneously. (Feuerstein 1998, p. 253)

The Yoga Sutras of Patanjali were dated to around 200 C.E. and gave yoga its classical format (see "The Eight Limbs of Yoga").

Western interest in yoga began about 150 years ago (Carrico 1997). Members of the Concord circle, such as Ralph Waldo Emerson and Henry David Thoreau, were inspired by the Bhagavad Gita. They shared their interest for this exotic philosophy with a small group of like-minded people. In 1877 Helene Blavatsky, a Russian emigré and occultist, published *Isis Unveiled* and in 1888 published *The Secret Doctrine*, works that divulged many of the ancient Vedic texts.

In 1893, Swami Vivekananda appeared before the World Parliament of Religions in Chicago, where he lectured on the merits of raja yoga (the yoga of meditation). In 1899 he returned to the United States and founded the New York Vedanta Society, a community that continues today, teaching raja, karma, bhakti, and jnana yoga. For the next 30 years yoga remained known and was practiced mainly for its philosophical aspects. In 1919 Yogendra Mastamani came to New York and demonstrated the power of hatha yoga to Americans. His own guru, Paramahansa Madhavadasaji, had been instrumental in reviving hatha yoga as a physical culture throughout India at the turn of the century. Another of Madhavadasaji's students, Kuvalayananda, had been encouraged to create the Kaivalyadhama Ashram and Research Institute near Pune, India, where physicians and scientists could study the more scientific aspects of hatha yoga. In 1922, Mastamani founded the first American branch of Kaivalyadhama and began a dialogue with the American medical community—particularly the alternative physicians of the time—thus establishing yoga as a viable healing therapy. His relationship with Benedict Lust, founder of naturopathy, began a relationship between yoga and alternative medicine healing practices that continues today.

In 1920 Paramahansa Yogananda came to Boston, where he addressed the International Congress of Religious Liberals. After a 3-year tenure in Boston, he toured the United States and, in 1925, founded the Self Realization Fellowship in Los Angeles, which has since attracted hundreds of thousands of followers and remains a strong force in the yoga community today. In 1947 Indra Devi, who studied hatha yoga with Krishnamacharya in India for several years, opened her own yoga studio in Hollywood, California. She taught thousands of students and trained hundreds of teachers. Among her clients were Hollywood celebrities Jennifer Jones, Gloria Swanson, and Robert Ryan, who helped to bring the benefits of hatha yoga to the public's attention.

With the advent of television and a more body-oriented culture, hatha yoga began to spread quickly. Richard Hittleman (1969) and Lilias Folan (1976) began to practice yoga before television audiences all over America. Hittleman's book, *The 28-Day Yoga Plan*, sold millions of copies.

In the 1960s and 1970s, many people began to turn to meditation in the spirit of searching for meaning and new values. This movement was publicized around the world when the Beatles visited India and were initiated into Maharishi Mahesh Yogi's Transcendental Meditation. Around the same time, Ram Dass published *Be Here Now* and established meditation in the public mind. Since the 1970s, hatha yoga has continued to flourish and diversify with the arrival of several great teachers from India, among them B. K. S. Iyengar, Yogi Bhajan, Swami Vishnu-devananda, and Pattabhi Jois.

Obstacles to the Use of Yoga in Western Medicine

The U.S. National Institutes of Health (NIH) Office of Alternative Medicine noted that "thousands of research studies" have shown that people can learn to control "physiological parameters" with yoga. Yet very few efficacy studies are under way (Morris 1998). A MEDLINE search with the heading "yoga" resulted in 421 items, but the vast majority of these are case reports, small studies, and anecdotal reports. Of the 421 items found, fewer than 10 report on the injuries or negative effects secondary to yogic practices. Most publications report positive results in a wide variety of conditions. This can be said of very few other medical treatments. This apparently highly effective treatment modality continues to exist on the fringes of Western medicine. It is more often patients who seek out alternative treatments when confronted with serious, chronic, or life-threatening illness; rarely does a health care provider actually prescribe yoga. One of the main reasons for this may be a lack of general knowledge about yoga on the part of physicians.

The continuing paradigm clash between the consciousness disciplines and Western psychology and psychiatry is a second reason why yoga is not often used. Roger Walsh (1980) described the "consciousness disciplines" as a

> family of practices and philosophies of primarily Eastern origin. Their central claim is that through intensive mental training it is possible to obtain [higher] states of consciousness and psychological well-being . . . as well as [gain] profound insight into the nature of mental processes, consciousness, and reality. (pp. 663)

Walsh went on to argue that rather than Western and Eastern disciplines being categorically different paradigms, Eastern concepts can be understood as an extension or more complete representation of the possible levels of consciousness—a view shared by the school of transpersonal psychology (Wilber 1977, 1979). To adequately understand the consciousness disciplines requires an openness to the possibility that these systems of thought may be different from western conventions of thinking but are just as sophisticated. An obstacle to providing additional research is that studies will likely only be funded by nonprofit or government organizations.

A third difficulty in describing or fully understanding the nature of consciousness disciplines such as yoga is that these disciplines are experiential in nature. They elicit internal mental experiences and feeling states that are not fully captured in the verbal descriptions and communications of Western research. For some scientists, designing adequate studies may require training in both Eastern and Western disciplines.

A fourth problem affecting the use of yoga is that it requires consistent effort and practice on the part of the practitioner and patient before the desired result can be achieved. Yoga is an effective way to treat anxiety disorders, but the patient must study it for at least 6 weeks before improvement is measurable. In contrast, benzodiazepines work within an hour. This example highlights the change in attitude toward healing that is necessary if someone wishes to employ yogic practices. The patient must decide to be an active participant in order to become well.

Taking all of these difficulties into account, in this chapter I provide information about the essential philosophic and psychologic concepts of the yoga system and suggest guidelines that can be shared with patients interested in incorporating yoga into their health care regimen.

Philosophy of Yoga

The first lines of the yoga sutra attributed to Patanjali (translated by B. S. Miller 1996) are

1. This is the teaching of yoga.
2. Yoga is the cessation of the turnings of thought.
3. When thought ceases, the spirit stands in its true identity as observer to the world.
4. Otherwise, the observer identifies with the turnings of thought.

The sutra is the essential scripture of yoga, outlining the path to liberation as conceptualized by yoga philosophers. The teachings were transmitted orally from teacher to student until Patanjali compiled them around 200 C.E. The goal of yoga is liberation from the suffering of human existence. The phenomenal world is understood as a place of continuous suffering, where no experience other than the transcendence of the world itself is ultimately satisfying. The nature of the world is imperfect and impermanent, but recognition of this reality is avoided in the usual state of consciousness. All experiences either are painful or, if pleasurable, will again be experienced as painful because of their transience and ending. Liberation is only possible through escaping the cycle of experiences altogether.

The nature of the true self is inherently free, pure, and eternal. When in the embodied state in the course of countless reincarnations, the true self becomes embroiled with the imperfect world through mind and body and is continuously trying to satisfy cravings of the body and the mind, ignorant to the true state of the world. Desires are the cause for the attachment to the material world. The never-ending search for fulfillment of desires continues the delusion that this is the ultimate purpose of existence. Through embodiment, the true self assumes the burden of a physical body and mind that will sooner or later succumb to the laws of nature and decay and die. The egoic mind veils the true self from realizing the nature of the world. In the absence of a higher goal the mind continues to pursue all of its transient wishes and desires. As long as we remain engaged with the world through desire, thought, or action, we continue in the cycle of repeated rebirths.

The practice of yoga is a process of dehypnotization—the recognition of the everyday world as a delusion—leading to the realization that happiness can only be found in transcendence of the gross, physical world altogether, so that the true self can realize its pure, divine, and eternal nature. Meditation is the tool with which the mind is able to study itself, a torchlight of insight that the mind can turn on to view its own functioning. When awareness replaces unconsciousness, change can occur. The repeated practice of meditative absorption begins the undoing of unconscious impressions and karma created by the turning of thought in the mind. Unless all karma is resolved, the individual remains chained to an endless series of reincarnations.

Yoga accepts the reality of God, but the understanding of the nature of God has undergone different phases over the millennia. In the dualistic, older concept, God is separate and higher than matter and beings, a benevolent entity directing evolution and supporting the thrust of the true self toward freeing itself from the bondage of the world. Since the emergence of Tantra in the medieval ages, a more pantheistic concept has evolved in which this world is one of God's creations and his/her divinity shows through in every materialized object or being. Liberation can be achieved through the medium of body and mind without self-denying asceticism. There is a great chain of being in which everything is connected, from material forms on one end of the spectrum, through the subtle ground of nature, to the dimension of formless transcendental consciousness on the other end.

The world is a constant play of its male and female divine aspects: *Shiva*, the unmaterialized male spirit, and *Shakti*, the power and drive of creation through nature, the female aspect of the divine. The universe is without beginning, but the worlds have repeatedly gone through cycles of creation and destruction. According to yoga philosophy we are currently in the Dark Ages, where sloth, torpor, and amorality reign and true seekers are rare.

Every object, being, or thought in the universe (*prakriti*) except the divine self (*purusa*) is characterized by the three *gunas*, the three qualities: 1) *tamas*: the inertia of matter, laziness; 2) *rajas*: drive, motivation, restlessness; and 3) *sattva*: purity, illumination. The changing balances of these three qualities determine the momentary state. This concept is crucial to understanding Ayurvedic or Indian medicine, which diagnoses illnesses according to imbalances of the gunas and prescribes measures to reestablish their balances and increase sattva.

The path of yoga begins at the point at which most human beings exist according to yoga. For the mind to be able to meditate, or study itself, morally and ethically correct living must occur. Without this, more and more negative karma will be created and the bondage to the world will be intensified. The psychophysical entity of the body and emotions must be controlled and quieted through the practice of postures, pranayama (breath work), and pratyahara (sense withdrawal) to decrease interference and distractibility and to establish a climate in which the mind can be stilled. Every aspect of life becomes a part of this evolution, and once the necessary foundation for a more spiritually inspired existence has been laid, the practitioner embarks on the project of "changing his mind," the adventure of meditation.

Psychology of Yoga

The ultimate source of human suffering originates in the errone-ous belief in an individual body-mind, separate from all others. Liberation from suffering is the process of loosening the attach-ment to the individual ego (body-mind) and realizing the identi-fication with the transcendental self. Bondage and unhappiness persist as long as happiness is measured in individual gains and losses. The way to freedom is the practice of equanimity and the process of learning to become detached from the result of our ac-tions. Yoga understands the mind as a purely material object, a sense organ like the eyes or the ears, therefore obeying the laws of matter. In its usual unconscious state, the mind is primarily affected by the constant activity of the external world. It needs to be retrained slowly through meditation to respond more to the needs of the eternal, transcendental Self.

In our ever-changing world, we spend most of our energy try-ing to hold on to pleasure and to avoid pain. This naturally leads to frustration, because it is ultimately impossible to permanently exclude the negative spectrum of experience. During repeated meditation the yogin gains insight into the true nature of reality and observes the egoic mind and its restless, ever-changing moods. This has profound consequences for the experience of the phenomenal world in the present moment. Current existence is acutely experienced as being transient and the world as a play of constant beginning and cessation. Emotional reactivity is reduced, and all stimuli are experienced as passing. Suffering is less in-tensely felt; its power fades before the eternal backdrop of the all-encompassing Spirit.

Yoga postulates three levels of consciousness. The first is that of dreams, hallucinations, sleep, and illusion. It is completely un-conscious and devoid of accurate perception of reality. The second level is that of our everyday consciousness, which is able to per-ceive the nature of the material world correctly but is completely ignorant of the true nature of reality. Only in the third and highest level of consciousness is the individual open and able to perceive the true nature of the world and realize enlightenment/liberation. Yoga practice is designed to encourage development from level two to level three of consciousness. To benefit from yoga, the mind must be able to accurately perceive the nature of everyday, material reality. Yoga is not a treatment for severe psychopathology.

If our desires get frustrated or we experience pain, our whole system reacts with stress. The body functions in fight–flight pattern, and suboptimal patterns of pain avoidance may be formed. In yoga psychology, detachment from the fluctuations of everyday existence is systematically practiced and thereby the physiologic reactivity to any given external or internal stimuli is reduced. This is accomplished through the steps of the eight-limb path: the physical postures increase control over voluntary muscles and work off stress hormones accumulated in the body. Pranayama, or breathing exercises, improve control over the autonomic system. Pratyahara, or sense withdrawal, practices intentional reduction of sensory stimuli and concentration. Meditation is used to reexamine thought patterns and to increase self-awareness and insight into neurotic patterns and habits. These patterns and habits, if left unexamined, are repeated unconsciously. The practitioner heightens the ability to voluntarily control action toward a healthier goal.

All of these practices take place in a milieu of increased relaxation, because all of the above-mentioned maneuvers will foster a physiologic response of relaxation (Wilber et al. 1986). In a more relaxed state it becomes increasingly possible to examine a situation rationally and choose the best possible response rather than react instinctually or habitually. Yoga philosophy teaches that everyone and everything in this universe is of the same essence and therefore inherently "good enough." Identification with our essence is fostered instead of the habitual identification with the transient expression of the ego. If the degree of attachment to the result of our actions is decreased, so is the danger of self-denigrating judgment for yet another perceived failure, which positively influences self-esteem.

With reduced attachment to results, the degree of self-control is thus increased and unrealistic expectations of oneself or the environment are reexamined and modified. A more realistic and less emotionally charged assessment of the environment allows the undoing of projections and other defensive perceptions. The degree of paranoia toward and perceived threat from the environment lessens, thus allowing an increase in free and creative expression. Yoga considers the mind to be one of the senses. Yoga differentiates between three parts of the mind: the lower mind (*manas*), the ego (*ahamkara*, the I-maker), and the critical, rational, decision-making faculty of the higher mind (*buddhi*). Beyond this lies the Self—the transcendental, divine, unchanging, and eternal essence of every living being.

The purpose of the lower mind is to manage sensory input, instincts, and drives and ensure basic survival. The more primitive the state of development, the more a being is chained to an automatic, instinctual way of reacting. Animals as well as children are dominated by this level of functioning. The purpose of mental development is to increase and widen the influence of the higher mind (buddhi), which is able to react independently of instinctual urges, to weigh the pros and cons rationally, and to act in ethical ways that will benefit the individual and society in the long run. The ego, or I-maker, is conceptualized very differently from Western psychology. The main function of the I-maker is to give a subjective interpretation to a given sense impression, for example, "the grass is green" becomes "I see green grass." It does not have a negotiating function between the other aspects of mind. It defines the transient traits of identity but distracts and deludes from the essence of the true self.

Yoga psychology does not explore early childhood development or the steps necessary for the establishment of a competent ego able to negotiate everyday reality. Yoga and other meditative psychologies do not aim at undoing healthy functioning in the world in favor of a reunion with a fantasized mystical ur-state of cosmic primordial oneness (Wilber et al. 1986). Rather, they favor a continuation of mental development beyond the "reasonably well-adjusted rational human being" and proclaim the existence of higher stages of spiritual development. Wilber and colleagues (1986) warn of confusing these higher stages of development with primitive ego states because both states are nonrational (pre/trans fallacy), or of reducing samadhi, which is the state of meditative ecstasy, to an autistic, symbiotic, undifferentiated state of early development. Atman, the one universal Self, is not the monadic-autistic self.

Yoga postulates the modern notion of an unconscious, vast and larger than the conscious mind, where all imprints of anything we do, will, or think are stored and determine further action and faith if left unexamined. "Every experience leaves its impress on the psyche, or mind. Ego-derived experiences reinforce the ego-illusion, whereas moments of self-transcendence in daily life or in the ecstatic state strengthen the spiritual impulse" (Feuerstein 1998, p. 320). Subliminal activators determine psychomental activity in the conscious mind and in our actions and faith. Unless the unconscious content is completely transcended through repeated practice of supraconscious ecstasy during meditation, we remain trapped in the circle of our karmic faith. Sri Aurobindo, modern-day Indian sage and philosopher, wrote: "It is true that the subliminal in man is the largest part of his nature and has in it the secret of the unseen dynamisms which explain his surface activities" (Aurobindo 1993, p. 265) He criticizes psychoanalysis for focusing primarily on the "lower vital subconscious" of instinctual drives and neglecting the higher levels of the unconscious, including the superconscience, which extends to the higher planes of mental being and the spiritual realms. He believed that to "purify and transform nature, it is the power of these higher ranges to which one must open and raise to them and change by them both the subliminal and the surface being" (p. 265). He warned that to focus on the lower levels of the subconscious prematurely was to risk everything foul and obscure to come to the surface without the guiding light of a strong and firm higher mind. Real and successful change is possible if this sequence is followed.

Like psychoanalysis and the psychotherapies, yoga aspires toward better adjustment to reality. However, it differs in its perception of the nature of reality and the path to the goal.

The Eight Limbs of Yoga

Yama

No spiritual accomplishment is possible without ethical and moral standards of living. Yoga follows the universal practices of nonviolence (*ahimsa*), truthfulness (*satya*), nonstealing (*asteya*), chastity (*brahmacharya*), and greedlessness (*aparigraha*). It is worth examining the meaning of these terms in a little more detail, because they illustrate the underlying unifying concept.

Ahimsa. Ahimsa is the practice of complete abstinence from violent action, motivation, or thought toward any living being, oneself, or the environment. For example, it would go against the principle of nonviolence and noninjury to exercise one's body during a fever or to pollute the environment with which we are intimately connected. Nonviolence extends to avoiding hateful thoughts and anger toward others or oneself.

Satya. Satya is truthfulness, without which living is inauthentic and will never allow for spiritual practice.

Asteya. Asteya is the practice of nonstealing. Stealing from others is meant in the broadest sense, including the unauthorized appropriation of things as well as the stealing of ideas or thoughts not belonging to oneself.

Brahmacharya. Brahmacharya is sexual abstinence in deed, words, or thought. This is considered essential because sexual stimulation is thought to weaken the impulse toward spiritual practice and enlightenment by satisfying immediate sensory experience and maintaining the status quo. (Tantric schools have embraced sexuality and devised elaborate rituals to channel the vital energy of sex [*ojas*] in the service of spiritual growth; see Hatha Yoga Pradipika 1985.) The rules are more relaxed for married yogis. Abstinence is said to increase the amount of energy and vigor at one's disposal for higher purpose.

Aparigraha. Aparigraha includes contentment with one's material possessions and the nonacceptance of gifts that will only cause attachments and distractions for the mind, thus chaining the person to this current existence. Some later yoga texts mention compassion, uprightness, patience, steadfastness, and a sparing (vegetarian) diet as additional moral precepts. It is understood that to achieve perfection in any of these precepts requires long and conscientious practice but that mastery of them will procure certain paranormal powers (*siddhis*). The moral precepts (*yama*) regulate and harmonize social interactions.

Niyama

The five practices of niyama are the basic rules for personal conduct that regulate the practitioner's relationship to life at large and harmonize his or her inner life.

Shauca (Purity)

Purification is a key metaphor of yogic spirituality and has a twofold meaning. In one aspect, purification means external cleanliness, including baths, special yogic cleanings (*kriya*), and a proper (vegetarian) diet. The other aspect refers to internal purity, which is achieved by concentration and meditation.

Samtosha (Contentment)

Contentment means not wanting more than one has. Indifference toward material possessions is the practice that will later allow equanimity in the face of pleasure or sorrow, success or failure. It is voluntary sacrifice of what will be relinquished anyway at the moment of death.

Tapas (Austerity)

Ascetic practices include fasting, prolonged immobilized sitting, bearing of hunger and thirst, and practice of postures to generate great psychosomatic energy and fuel for higher spiritual awareness. The literal translation of tapas is "heat," the spiritual fire created by nonindulgence. It does not mean self-castigation or denial of basic needs that would cause *himsa* (violence, harm).

Svadhyaya (Study)

Svadhyaya refers to the learning and absorption of the ancient wisdom and study of the scriptures of yoga. The integration of the knowledge into the mind and the meditative pondering of the teachings are considered an essential tool in the process of abolishing dysfunctional mind habits.

Ishvara-Pranidhana (Devotion to the Lord)

Devotion to the Lord is "the heart opening to the transcendental Being who for the unenlightened individual is an objective reality and force, but who upon enlightenment is found to coincide with the yogin's transcendental self" (Feuerstein 1998, p. 329).

Asana

The practice of postures continues the process of turning inward that was begun with the ethical disciplines and that now turns the focus onto the body. The practice of postures serves to improve physical health, sharpen internal awareness, and prepare the body for the rigors of extended meditation. It also serves to prepare the body for the onslaught of energy that will occur when the Kundalini energy is awakened (Kundalini or Laya yoga). Yogic postures are said to purify the body and eliminate toxins.

There are between 85 and 250 yoga postures (asanas) said to be beneficial for the human body. The asanas are a form of calisthenic exercise, more or less rigorous depending on the particular school and level of the student. Postures need to be learned from a teacher to avoid injury and to learn the anatomically correct form. They will improve strength, balance, and flexibility. Regular daily practice is encouraged for increased benefits; the typical length of practice is between 30 and 105 minutes. Movements are slow and never forced beyond the practitioner's ability. Pain is avoided and is a sign to stop. At the same time, a slow extension of the boundaries of strength and flexibility is encouraged and is achieved by the regular repetition of a particular posture. In a complete departure from most Western exercise, yoga can be practiced only in a noncompetitive environment, which for most beginners is the most difficult aspect to grasp. When asanas are practiced in a competitive spirit, they are likely to lead to injury. Postures are balanced—always practiced symmetrically and in combination with particular counterposes to avoid strain. They are beneficial for deep tissues and inner organs as well, increasing circulation and perfusion and encouraging the elimination of waste products. Certain postures are designed to temporarily reduce or increase blood flow to a particular organ and massage and stimulate its functioning. The postures are a relatively low-impact exercise, thus allowing the practitioner to feel more relaxed, alert, and refreshed at the end of practice. Aerobic muscle metabolism is maintained throughout the practice. Figure 3–1 provides some examples of yoga postures.

Pranayama

Pranayama literally translates as "life force extension" and refers to bioenergy, or prana, that infuses and sustains life according to yoga philosophy. Yogic practices aim at freeing energy blocks, increasing prana, and directing it for the purpose of spiritual progress. Ordinarily involuntary processes can become more accessible to voluntary control.

Prana's external manifestation is the breath. Controlling the breath allows direct influence over the internal milieu and can help regulate emotional states and the mind. Several different breathing techniques are practiced. The basic yogic breath is a full diaphragmatic breath that perfuses the whole lung and increases breathing capacity. Kapalabhati breathing, the rapid alternation of forced exhalation and passive inhalation, is used as a cleansing exercise.

Alternate nostril breathing is practiced by temporarily blocking off one nostril, thus slowing down the rate of breath and improving oxygenation. Postures are often practiced in the rhythm of another breathing technique, ujjayi, in which the throat is partially closed through muscular effort, causing a snoring-like sound and again improving oxygenation. Other therapeutic breathing exercises, shitali and shitakari, are considered cooling exercises and are performed by bending the tongue to form a roll and breathing through the resulting spaces. Beyond these commonly used techniques several other breathing practices are used.

When these four stages have been mastered, the yogin is prepared to turn the focus to the mind and meditation. The transition is completed by the fifth of the eight limbs, *pratyahara*.

Pratyahara

With pratyahara, the process of desensitization to external stimuli that was begun with the practice of postures and breath control

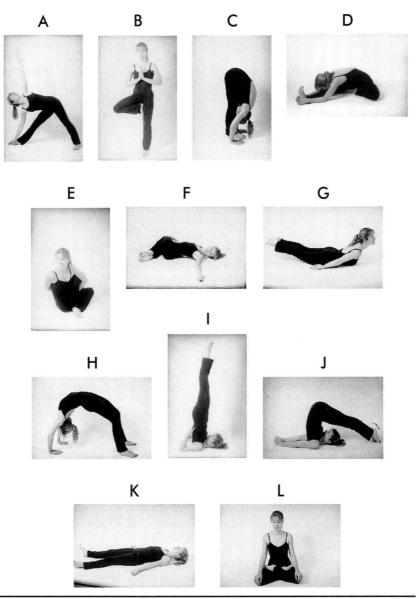

Figure 3–1. Examples of yoga postures.

These photos are not meant as instructional guides. Standing poses: triangle (**A**) and tree pose (**B**). Forward bends: standing forward bend (**C**) and janusirsasana (**D**). Twists: sitting twist (**E**) and lying twist (**F**). Backbends: lying boat pose (**G**) and wheel pose (**H**). Inversions: shoulderstand (**I**) and plow pose (**J**). Relaxation and meditation poses: savasana (corpse pose) (**K**) and lotus pose (**L**).

is now made the focus of the practice. The attention is withdrawn from the senses one by one, and sensory input is minimized. Focus now turns entirely to the inner environment of the mind.

Dharana

Concentration (*dharana*) trains the mind to be one-pointed, with full attention on a single object. When distractions from the external environment have been minimized, the practitioner's attention turns to the ongoing flow of thoughts, the constant distracted chatter of the mind, and attempts to stabilize attention on a single object, usually a part of the body (chakra), the internalized image of an external object (e.g., deity), or a sacred sound (mantra). Once mastered, dharana is different from purely intellectual concentration in that it is more powerful but effortless at the same time.

Dyana

Prolonged and deepening concentration slowly leads to meditation (*dyana*), in which the object of concentration fills the entire space of consciousness. Arising thoughts no longer elicit an emotional response because the external environment is effectively blocked out. There is an increase in lucidity and wakefulness, and at the same time a complete absence of restlessness or everyday concerns.

Samadhi

Samadhi, or ecstasy, ensues when all impressions and mental fluctuations have been fully resolved through intensive meditation. It has been described as a complete merging of the subjective consciousness with the object. This identification is accompanied by a widening of consciousness and the experience of bliss and peacefulness. Patanjali differentiated between conscious ecstasy and supraconscious ecstasy, with conscious ecstasy possessing four subcategories. The essence of conscious ecstasy is the partial, transient transcendence of the ego-personality.

In supraconscious ecstasy, the fusion occurs with the transcendental, divine Self. It is described as the only way to recover conscious awareness of the transcendental Self. When this state of ecstasy is maintained over sufficiently long periods, the subliminal activators are slowly obliterated and the resultant karma is avoided. This union of individual existence with the true self is the goal of yoga and the endpoint of practice—liberation. For Patanjali, this moment coincided with the shedding (i.e., death) of the individual body-mind and the abiding as an attribute-less Self in unmanifest realms. Other writers maintained that this state of *nirvikalpa samadhi* could be entered into and left, repeatedly, during this lifetime (Hatha Yoga Pradipika 1985).

Yoga in Health and Prevention

The practice of yoga leads to an increased sense of wholeness and centeredness of experience. This decreases the amount of time spent in mental reevaluation of the past or in planning for the future. The result is a heightened sense of presence and intensity of experience in the current moment. There is a change in the person's outlook and less restriction in the choice of behavior. Because the individual is understood as a piece of an interconnected whole, the perception of the "outside" world changes as well. If there is no outside, there is no necessity for suspicion or fear of the other, thus allowing for more fulfilling relationships. An important part of the social aspect of these teachings is the idea of compassion and altruism toward others; through good deeds there is a creation of good karma. Interconnectedness meditations are practiced to become more other-focused, which is said to increase personal happiness.

Although physical and mental wellness are only side effects of the true yogic goal, they are potent reinforcers for continued practice. Yoga would not have survived the millennia and achieved its current degree of support in the West if the only benefit was the promise of liberation in the distant future. It provides us with a map for a lifestyle change toward greater health and introduces the tools in pragmatic ways, thereby accentuating our responsibility toward ourselves. Yoga is an ideal tool for illness prevention, with recommendations for the right diet, physical activity, stress reduction, and group support.

Yoga has adapted to the West and has changed significantly over the last century. This is demonstrated by the blossoming of hatha yoga (the physical, forceful practice of postures). This branch of yoga was nearly extinct in India at the turn of the century. It was revived through export to the West and the creativity of a number of twentieth-century teachers. Adapting to Western needs, it has become accessible to a large number of people, has become more tangible, and is now less of an obscure, occult science. For the purpose of wellness, yoga can and should be practiced without religious connotations because its benefits are independent of religious orientation and practices.

Probably the largest area of potential benefit for yogic practices is for improved wellness and primary prevention. Yoga promotes a healthy lifestyle that encompasses every aspect of existence. A person who decides to practice yoga should spend between 20 minutes and 2 hours each day practicing postures, breathing exercises, and meditation. This demanding schedule will probably prevent yoga from becoming part of the average American's lifestyle. On the other hand, elements of its teachings, predominantly the physical aspects, have been integrated into physical therapy, prebirthing classes, and forms of exercise such as pilates and athletic cross-training. The practice of physical postures has been gaining momentum in certain subgroups of the population, such as seniors and pregnant women. The gentle nature of the exercises allows its use in almost any condition. Yoga therapists are adapting the postures even for bed-bound patients.

Over the past 20 years, several studies have been performed to study the effects of yoga in healthy people. The consensus seems to be that it has an overall beneficial effect with a very positive effect on mood: hatha yoga was superior to other exercise in increasing life satisfaction, alertness, enthusiasm, high spirits, extravertedness, and perception of mental and physical energy. Yoga students also exhibited decreased scores in excitability, aggressiveness, somatic complaints, anger, and tension. Their ability to cope with stress was significantly better (Berger and Owen 1992; Schell 1994; Wood 1993).

Yoga has been shown to improve exercise tolerance, cognitive performance, and respiratory and cardiac parameters. In an Indian study, Raju et al. (1997) examined the short-term effects of 4 weeks of intensive yoga training on the exercise tolerance (treadmill) of healthy volunteers. Results showed a 21% increase in maximal work output with a significantly reduced level of oxygen consumption per unit work, but without a significant change in heart rate. Subjects were able to exercise more comfortably, with a significantly lower heart rate, reduced minute ventilation, and a significantly lower respiratory quotient. Madanmohan et al. (1992) found that a 12-week practice of yoga led to a significant reduction in auditory and visual reaction times, significantly increased breath holding times, and increased respiratory pressures.

These are some examples of the various benefits that could be expected if more studies were available. The studies support the subjective experience of yoga students who report an increase in mental and physical energy, improved exercise tolerance and stamina, better mood, and improved relationships. Concentration is improved and joy can be derived from a much wider variety of events than before. The commitment to a healthier lifestyle increases: practitioners often decide to quit smoking or drinking alcohol, eat healthier diets, and reduce the amount of stress in their daily lives.

Yoga and Psychiatry

The very detailed psychology of yoga invites application in psychiatry, although research is still largely lacking. Thus far, the available data suggest a mood-enhancing effect and decreased levels of anxiety as the result of the use of yogic techniques. The most thorough data on the use of the yogic techniques of postures, breathing, and meditation stem from a two-part Indian study (Vahia et al. 1966, 1973). In the pilot study, 30 patients with psychosomatic and psychiatric disturbances were taught standard yogic practices for 4–6 weeks. The biggest problem during the study was that 13 patients were lost to follow-up. The highest rates of success were seen with patients diagnosed with "anxiety reaction": 6 of 14 were significantly improved. Two patients with schizophrenia who participated in the study were advised to discontinue the yoga treatment. This study highlights some of the difficulties in performing research on yogic techniques. It is practically impossible to standardize the content of what is taught to patients, and even if it were possible, the fact that yoga is given in the form of instruction from teacher to student introduces the human element as a bias. Furthermore, any protocol using yoga techniques is bound to produce a high dropout rate considering the amount of effort that is required on the part of study participants. Researchers are left with a self-selected group of people with higher degrees of will, determination, and perseverance, elements that affect prognosis. Of the 95 patients who participated in the main study, 73% in the yoga group showed an improvement of at least 50%, whereas only 42% in the control group showed such a significant improvement. On the Taylor anxiety scale the yoga group showed a significantly greater reduction in anxiety than the control group. Similar results were obtained on the Minnesota Multiphasic Personality Inventory scores of both groups. Within the yoga group, subjects who displayed greater skill in meditation showed more clinical improvement.

Yoga psychology contains elements of several Western therapies, including biofeedback, supportive and group therapy, and insight-oriented as well as cognitive-behavioral therapy (CBT). Extending beyond the purely psychologic level, it has significant physiologic effects (in India it has been called *psychophysiological therapy*). There is no Western psychotherapy that pays the same degree of attention to physiologic parameters or to integrating mind and matter. The more body-oriented therapies, such as Gestalt therapy or bioenergetics, use the body mainly for diagnostic purposes. CBT teaches relaxation skills but in a less thorough way (i.e., during a hatha yoga class, the entire practice will stimulate the physiology of relaxation). Yoga has features of psychodynamic psychotherapy in that it acknowledges the central importance of a self and an unconscious. It aims at increased self-awareness and sees most behavior as determined by unconscious motivation. Symptoms are viewed as originating in unconscious, maladaptive conflict solutions, and the goal of therapy is the undoing of the original conflict, not just symptom relief. Integration of the human personality is the desired goal.

Yoga differs from psychodynamic therapy in many important ways. A transference relationship with the teacher is not necessary and not encouraged for the process (although it may occur). A second important difference is the definition of traumatic conflict: psychoanalytic therapies view neurotic symptom formation as suboptimal conflict resolution for the purpose of reducing anxiety in the psychic system. Conflict arises between psychic structures (id, ego, superego). In yoga psychology the onset of conflict is perceived to arise from a faulty perception and evaluation of the nature of reality and the relationship between the individual and reality. In contrast to psychoanalysis, yoga postulates a third and highest level of consciousness that can be achieved through the yogic method (i.e., meditation). This is the level of the superconscious (Aurobindo 1995). There is no equivalent to this level of consciousness in Western psychology. Psychoanalytic concepts are devoid of spiritual ideas. In yoga they are part of the essence. Yoga embraces them and establishes spiritual accomplishment as a worthwhile life goal. The nature of the unconscious differs substantially in both systems. According to Freud, only socially forbidden desires and unacceptable drives are pushed into the unconscious to allow functioning in the everyday world. In yoga, all thoughts or activities will leave unconscious traits and continue the ego-attachment. Meditative purification and stopping of the thoughts are the only tools that will facilitate decreased unconscious activity. The main tool in this process is to attempt to achieve a high level of one-pointed concentration that permits the exclusion of everyday activity and thought in the service of the goal of "refinding" the true transcendental self. The tool of psychoanalysis is free association, that is, an encouragement for increased, uncensored, nondirected activity of thought in the service of unearthing of unconscious material so it is available for analysis and integration.

Drives are important determinants for action in both traditions. Psychoanalysis advocates a sublimation of drives toward a higher purpose. The ascetic schools of yoga recommend a reduction or restraining of the drives, especially the sex drive, which is perceived as a hindrance on the spiritual path. The energy that gets dispersed through sex would otherwise be available for spiritual pursuits. Tantric schools of yoga devised a process to deal with drives that more closely resembles sublimation. In tantra, scholars attempt to experience the pleasures of this world, because the pleasures as well as everything else in this world are essentially expressions of the divine. The energy released with the drive can then be channeled in the service of spiritual accomplishment. In the example of the sexual drive, sexual activity in tantra is highly ritualized. One must follow the prescribed rituals to salvage the sexual energies and transform them into spiritual energy for the purpose of liberation.

The last and most important difference is that yoga was devised as a system for higher mental development to be carried out by mentally healthy individuals, whereas psychoanalysis is a treatment for psychiatric pathology. All application of yoga and other consciousness psychologies must therefore be applied with extreme care for patients with severe character pathology. Little information is available to guide the use of yoga other than anecdotal descriptions of negative outcomes.

Some psychotherapists have been carefully introducing Eastern ideas for use in psychodynamic psychotherapy. Epstein (1998) described his journey as a therapist and meditator and gave several examples of how he infused his practice of psychotherapy with ideas derived from Buddhist psychology, which shares many ideas with yoga psychology. He discussed the questionable value of ever firmer and more impenetrable ego boundaries, an idea celebrated in Western psychology (pp. 84–85). Buddhist and yoga psychology emphasize the value of intermittently relaxing the otherwise intact ego boundaries to allow increased connectedness and authenticity of experience. This opening to the world does not have to be pathologic as long as it occurs within a healthy ego and is then a form of adaptation. For example, during love and play the boundaries need to be relaxed so that a temporary merging with another or with an object can occur and deep experience is possible.

Yoga psychology resembles CBT in that it introduces a method for systematic retraining and relearning for the mind and gives clear prescriptions for behavior modification. In contrast with CBT, yoga does not stay within the paradigm of avoiding pain and increasing pleasurable experiences, but tries to transcend the paradigm toward a state of equanimity beyond pain or pleasure. Yoga encourages focusing on pain or a painful stimulus instead of avoidance as long as it occurs in the context of detached, open, and discriminative attention that allows the exploration of the nature of the stimulus. Through meditation and relaxation techniques, the practitioner is more able to continue the use of detached attention and reduce emotional reactivity.

Yoga involves elements of supportive psychotherapy, including giving advice, direction, encouragement, and reassurance. The teacher is an expert working to help the student's development and is nonjudgmental. Classes are taken frequently (weekly to daily), usually in the same room, and are paid for. Like psychotherapy, yoga claims to be useful, thereby potentially eliciting the placebo effect. Because yoga is often practiced in a group environment, it encourages group support and peer relationships and thus adds an interpersonal, social element.

Since yoga arrived in the West, thinkers and therapists have tried to understand, integrate, or use yoga therapeutically in conjunction with Western psychology. Jung was the first prominent psychiatrist to become interested in yoga. He gave a series of seminars in 1932 comparing the chakra system of Kundalini yoga with Western psychologic concepts (Jung 1996). He began with the assumption that Western psychology was superior to its Eastern counterpart and that Westerners would not be able to truly benefit from this Eastern technology because of cultural differences. He therefore did not adequately give justice to the sophistication of the model of the chakras and their symbolism. In 1990, Rama et al. published *Yoga and Psychotherapy: the Evolution of Consciousness*, which more thoroughly and neutrally explained key concepts of yoga psychology for Western readers.

Psychiatric Indications for Yoga

Yogic techniques have been applied successfully as an adjuvant therapy to many more disorders than mentioned in the following paragraphs. Readers interested in further information are referred to the following resources from the yoga literature: Iyengar

1979; Jois 1999; Monro et al. 1990; Sharma and Singh 1997; Shivapremananda 1997; and Weller 1995.

Anxiety Disorders

Yogic postures, breathing exercises, and beginning stages of meditation foster a state of relaxation that is helpful in reducing levels of general anxiety and worry. They reduce blood pressure and pulse, eliciting the relaxation response. The cognitive process of outlook and habit change alter perception of reality from a threatening entity toward a more benign world and allow reevaluation of the perceived threat in a more realistic way. J. J. Miller et al. (1995) teaches stress reduction through the use of mindfulness meditation, yogic postures, and relaxation techniques to medical patients at the University of Massachusetts Medical Center. In a 3-year follow-up to this 8-week training course, 22 medical patients with anxiety disorders as defined by DSM-III-R (American Psychiatric Association 1987) were investigated. There were clinically and statistically significant improvements in subjective and objective symptoms of anxiety and panic following the initial intervention. Of the original subjects, 18 were available for a 3-year follow-up. The majority of subjects had been compliant with the meditation practice at the time of follow-up. Repeated measures analysis showed maintenance of the gains obtained in the original study on the Hamilton and Beck anxiety and depression scales. Improvement was maintained as well on the Hamilton panic score, the number and severity of panic attacks, and on the Mobility Index–Accompanied and the Fear Survey.

Vahia et al. (1973) used psychophysical therapy (which follows the eight-limb path of raja yoga) to treat neurotic and psychosomatic disorders (anxiety, depression, hysteria, asthma). They found that this yoga therapy was effective.

Yoga sources prescribe relaxation, meditation, pranayama (especially victorious breath and alternate nostril breathing), asanas, (especially corpse pose and shoulder stand), reappraisal of lifestyle, and avoidance of coffee, cigarettes, and alcohol. For panic attacks, awareness of the symptom "anxiety" and presence to the symptom during an attack is recommended together with the practice of relaxation after a panic attack. Physical postures should be practiced regularly with a focus on the shoulder-stand sequence and breathing exercises that slow down the rate of breathing and increase oxygenation (kapalabhati and ujjayi).

Depression

The practice of postures, breathing exercises, and concentrative meditation induce a sense of well-being that may support conventional psychiatric treatment. Meditation can instill a sense of calm. Motivation and cooperation with regular practice may be stumbling blocks in the presence of more severe depression. Sudarshan kriya yoga (in which the focus is on meditation) is uniformly effective for depression of both the dysthymic and the melancholic type (Murthy 1998). Yogic prescriptions for mild depression include an active physical program of asanas to increase energy (sun salutations and backbends), pranayama (alternate nostril breathing, shitali, shitakari, and kapalabhati), and short periods spent in deep relaxation or meditation.

Obsessive-Compulsive Disorder

Yoga therapy prescribes alternate nostril breathing for treatment of obsessive-compulsive disorder (OCD). Shannahoff-Khalsa and Beckett (1996) from the University of California at San Diego provided some validation for efficacy of the ancient breathing technique for the treatment of OCD. Eight patients with OCD were taught unilateral forced nostril breathing and then practiced it for a year. Subjects showed a decrease in scores on the Yale-Brown Obsessive Compulsive Scale, with a mean improvement of 54%. The Symptom Checklist–90—Revised showed significant improvement comparing baseline to 12 months. Perceived Stress Scale scores showed significant improvement as well. Of five patients who had been stabilized on fluoxetine prior to the study, three stopped the medication after 7 months or less, and two significantly reduced its use. The authors concluded that these results warranted further study for the use of yoga in OCD, impulse control, and anxiety disorders.

Posttraumatic Stress Disorder

No research data are available for the use of yoga in treatment of posttraumatic stress disorder (PTSD). In the yoga literature, treatment focuses on relaxation and breathing techniques to benefit hyperarousal symptoms in acute PTSD. Breathing exercises should focus on lengthening the exhalation, which has calming effects. Depending on the presence of physical trauma, postures may be used as a restorative physical exercise under supervision of an experienced yoga therapist.

In PTSD due to sexual and physical abuse, yoga postures should be used with extreme caution because they may rekindle memories and flashbacks to the traumatic situation. After the trauma has been worked through in therapy, yoga may help to develop a more integrated body sense if practiced carefully with a sense of control and mastery.

Psychotic Disorders

Neither Western research nor yogic literature gives specific recommendations for the use of yogic techniques in psychotic disorders. In the presence of active psychosis, meditation is not possible. Yogic techniques other than physical postures should be practiced only under the guidance of an experienced teacher.

Personality Disorders

No research data are available for the use of yoga for personality disorders. Therefore, yoga should be used with care and as an adjunctive treatment. Several risks exist, including development of a transference relationship to the yoga teacher; misunderstanding of symptoms of the character disorder as achievements on the meditative path (e.g., borderline feelings of "emptiness" are mistaken for meditative stabilization); and resistance of change. Physical exercise (yoga asanas) and breathing techniques may be helpful for their relaxing properties and improved body sense. The treating psychotherapist should explore the effects of yogic practices with the patient and must be available to integrate those experiences into the goals of the therapy or, if necessary, warn in the face of impending disorganization.

Substance Abuse

A team at Harvard Medical School (Shaffer et al. 1997) compared methadone maintenance treatment enhanced by hatha yoga with dynamic group therapy. They found the hatha yoga program to be as effective as, but not more effective than, the dynamic group psychotherapy in a methadone program. Yoga psychology places significant importance on the breaking of addictive habits through insight and willpower of a trained mind. Cleansing breath (kapalabhati), mantra recitation, and vigorous practice of asanas interspersed with brief episodes of relaxation are recommended.

Chronic Insomnia

Regular practice of postures, breathing exercises, relaxation, and meditation will improve the quality of sleep.

Premenstrual Dysphoric Disorder and Menopause

Yoga therapy prescribes several postures to decrease symptoms of premenstrual dysphoric disorder and menopause: all seated poses, triangle pose, bow, and shoulder stand should be emphasized (see Figure 3–1 for demonstration of selected postures). Relaxation and meditation will have a positive effect.

Psychiatric Disturbances Caused by Yoga

The data are scarce and scattered regarding the psychiatric disturbances caused by yoga. Wilber et al. (1986) gave an excellent summary of the potential disturbances that may occur in the course of higher spiritual development. Problems befalling the beginner are related to inadequate understanding or practice of the teachings or identifications with certain aspects of them when unresolved pathologies remain from earlier stages of development. Some examples include psychic inflation, in which universal-transpersonal energies and insight are exclusively applied to the individual (remnants of narcissism interfere); psychotic episodes that occur when profound spiritual insights are channeled through a self structure that is neurotic, borderline, or psychotic;

the awakening of spiritual energies (Kundalini), which can have potentially dramatic consequences (Krishna 1972), altering completely the person's energetic state; and pranic disorders, in which Kundalini energy is misdirected through faulty technique. This may result in miscellaneous psychosomatic symptoms; yogic illness, in which the development of higher levels of consciousness puts undue strain on the physical–emotional body and causes physical disease; or, in advanced meditators, disturbances in the process of differentiation, separation, and transcendence of the previous level of development and disturbances in the process of integration and identification of the subtle archetypal self and its object relations.

Medical Indications for Yoga

Yoga has been studied as the sole or adjunct treatment in a wide variety of conditions, from sports injuries to medical illnesses such as heart disease, diabetes, and asthma. Overall, it has been found to be beneficial for most disorders studied, both objectively and subjectively. However, many reports of the benefits are still anecdotal, based on small samples or case reports. More rigorous studies are needed. In addition to the disorders mentioned below, yoga therapy recommends its practices in the following states or diseases: gastrointestinal disorders (irritable bowel syndrome, colitis, chronic constipation), sexual impotency, cervical and lumbar spondylitis, neuromuscular disorders, pregnancy, knee and other joint disorders, endocrine disorders, and urogenital disorders.

Hypertension

Sundar et al. (1984) studied the effects of savasana (yogic relaxation pose) performed by 25 patients with essential hypertension for 6 months. They found a statistically significant drop in systolic and diastolic blood pressures in patients both on and off antihypertensive medications. Patients who abandoned the practice of savasana after the study experienced a return to hypertension. Andrews et al. (1982) compared 37 reports of treatment of hypertension by nonpharmacologic means with the results of standard drug regimens. He found that a regimen of weight reduction, yoga, and relaxation led to a smaller but appreciable decrease in blood pressure compared with drug treatment. Yoga therapy recommends very gentle practice, using mainly relaxation poses, for more than mild hypertension. Alternate nostril breathing and ujjayi breath is taught, and the breath is never held, because this would increase intrathoracic pressure. Persons with hypertension should seek the help of an experienced yoga teacher and practice under supervision. Inverted poses (headstand, shoulder stand, standing forward bends) or poses that will increase the pressure in the chest must be avoided. Meditation is very valuable.

Heart Disease

Schmidt et al. (1997) examined cardiovascular risk factors and hormones during a comprehensive, residential, 3-month kriya yoga training and vegetarian nutrition study. They found a substantial risk factor reduction. Body mass index, total serum and low-density lipoprotein cholesterol, fibrinogen, and blood pressure were significantly reduced, especially in those with elevated levels at baseline. Urinary excretion of adrenaline, noradrenaline, dopamine, and aldosterone was reduced as were levels of serum testosterone and luteinizing hormone. Cortisol excretion increased significantly. Dean Ornish et al. (1979), with the help of Yogi Swami Satchidananda, developed a routine of physical postures as part of their program for reversing heart disease and attained positive results. Recommendations for yogic practice are the same as for hypertension. The focus is on relaxation. Backbending postures should be practiced very gently in patients with arrhythmias.

Asthma

The use of yogic postures, breathing techniques, and meditation for patients with asthma has been extensively studied (Goyeche et al. 1982; Jain et al. 1991; Khanam et al. 1996; Nagarathna 1998; Singh et al. 1990 [review]; Vedanthan et al. 1998). The definitive study was done by Nagendra and Nagarathna (1986). They followed up 570 bronchial asthmatic individuals for up to 54 months who had initially participated in a comprehensive training in yogic postures, breathing exercises, meditation, kriyas (cleansing techniques), and yogic theory. Results showed a highly significant improvement in most of the specific parameters, significantly decreased peak expiratory flow rate, and reduction in the use of medication. Yoga therapy aims at curing asthma; however, this will occur only with regular committed practice. Asanas strengthen chest muscles and remove energy blocks, inverted poses drain mucus from the lungs, breathing exercises improve respiratory functions, and meditation stabilizes the mind.

Seizures

Panjwani and colleagues (1996) found an 86% decrease in seizure frequency after 6 months of yogic meditation. Stancak and Kuna (1994) found that alternate nostril breathing has a balancing effect on the functional activity of the left and right hemisphere as shown on electroencephalogram (EEG). Yoga sources recommend a supportive role of yoga in the treatment of seizures. By increasing the degree of relaxation, stress and potential triggers of a seizure may be avoided. Jerking movements and kapalabhati breathing are to be avoided. Begin with meditation and breathing exercises and introduce postures slowly. Patients with prior yoga experience are encouraged to practice sun salutations (Jois 1999).

Ophthalmic Problems

For refraction problems, yogins practice a series of eye muscle exercises and relaxation. For detached retina and glaucoma, only breathing techniques (alternate nostril, ujjayi, shitali) are practiced. Inverted poses or breath-holding techniques that will increase the pressure in the eye should be avoided.

Back Pain

For back pain, yogic postures should be practiced slowly and in a balanced way to strengthen the truncal musculature evenly and increase flexibility of the spine without causing new imbalances or injuries to nerves and discs. Back and forward bends should be practiced cautiously after sufficient duration of practice (at least 1 month) without tightening the back muscles too much. Forward bends and twists are beneficial for muscle strain because they lengthen the spine and the space between the vertebrae. They should be avoided in the presence of disc problems. Relaxation and meditation (in a comfortable position) are highly recommended.

Obesity

Postures should be combined with a commitment for a lifestyle change including yogic diet (lactovegetarian). Monitor for increases in blood pressure and pulse during practice. Inverted postures must be avoided. All other postures may be practiced and are a gentle form of exercise for patients with sedentary habits. In yoga therapy, kapalabhati breathing is said to be beneficial to increase metabolism and further weight loss.

Headaches

Relaxation, meditation, and breathing exercises should be emphasized for headaches. If a diagnosis of tension headache is established, postures may be practiced because they can relieve muscular tension and strain. Patients with intracranial tumors, infarctions, or other such conditions may benefit from general relaxation. To be avoided are forward bends, inverted postures, and breath-holding techniques, all of which can increase intracranial pressure.

Patients Receiving Medications

There are no general contraindications to the use of medications with yoga. The practitioner should monitor and check medication side effects (e.g., orthostatic hypotension increases a risk of falling). The patient should avoid excessive forward and back bending.

Diabetes

Yoga appears to be beneficial for patients with diabetes. One study found a decrease in rates of hyperglycemia and hypoglycemia as well as in the need for oral hypoglycemic drugs after 40 days of training in yogic techniques (Jain et al. 1993). Yoga wisdom recommends asana practice for its supportive role with weight reduction and diet control. Postures focusing on the abdominal region (twists, back bends, bandhas) are said to improve the function of the pancreas.

Osteoarthritis, Rheumatoid Arthritis, Ankylosing Spondylitis, Fibromyalgia

Garfinkel and colleagues (1994, 1998) studied the use of a yoga-based exercise program in patients with osteoarthritis of the hands and carpal tunnel syndrome. They found that subjects in the yoga groups had significant improvement in grip strength, decreased pain during activity, decreased tenderness, and increased finger range of motion. Yoga therapy prescribes gentle and slow practice of postures combined with breathing and relaxation exercises.

Chronic Pain

Kabat-Zinn (1982) studied the effect of a 10-week training course in mindfulness meditation, yoga exercise, and relaxation techniques in patients with chronic pain. He concluded that mindfulness meditation led to a significant decrease in perceived pain and accompanying mood disturbances. Changes were relatively stable on follow-up. Yoga therapy for chronic pain is relaxation, meditation, and healing visualizations. Depending on the source and nature of the pain, yogic postures may help rehabilitation.

Injuries From Yogic Exercise

As with any physical activity, yogic exercise can lead to injury, especially when not performed correctly. There is remarkably little information on yoga-related injuries in the literature. The only reports stem from ophthalmology (retinal varices and detachments) and neurology (intracranial varices following extended headstands).

Conclusions

Although continued study of yoga with more sophisticated research designs is desirable, it can seem like trying to fit a square peg into a round hole. There can be little doubt that yogic techniques are more beneficial than harmful. It therefore seems indicated to use open trials to examine more claims made by yogis regarding the usefulness of yogic techniques for specific disorders. Another serious obstacle to studying yoga is the complexity of its interventions, which makes it almost impossible to control for unless restricted to a small population, thus contradicting the approach of yoga.

Yoga is inexpensive and readily available. It would be desirable if physicians could be guides to patients in this area so that Eastern and Western approaches to health could be combined for increased benefits. As a rule of thumb it is fair to say that yoga is generally recommendable as an adjunctive treatment, whereas the use of it as a sole treatment needs to be studied further.

Yoga's greatest potential contribution lies in the area of improving a sense of well-being in a healthy person or in someone who has a specific illness. Because the yoking of all elements of one's existence and experience induces an increased sense of well-being, this chance should not be forgone. With its demand to look at the true reality and to accept the current parameters that cannot be changed, yoga helps people reduce unrealistic expectations, accept current limitations, and improve the degree of happiness possible within the framework. The medical literature as well as yogic sources abound with case reports of people with a serious medical illness who have benefited from this tradition. This increasing evidence becomes very relevant in the face of increasing numbers of people who are living with chronic illnesses such as heart disease, cancer, or AIDS. Conventional medicine should continue to look for the cures; however, until such cures become available we should recommend ways of practice to our patients that make life happier and more meaningful.

Yoga practice is "too hard" and demanding to ever become mainstream, but it should be part of the momentum providing a strong enough impulse (together with other complementary techniques) for allopathic medicine and psychiatry to "yoke" the current compartmentalized approach to human beings and health.

It goes beyond the scope of this chapter to expand in detail on the ways in which yoga psychology could enrich the practice of psychiatry and medicine.

Similar to other physicians practicing alternative techniques in the framework of modern medicine, my interest in applying yoga to psychiatry stems from the remarkable results of my personal practice. In my work as a psychiatrist, it is my opinion that diagnosis and treatment have to consider traditional sources (DSM-IV [American Psychiatric Association 1994], psychodynamic understanding) as well as the whole web and network of interconnected and interrelated balances that make up an individual's complexity. As a therapist, I do not teach yoga or meditation, because this would blur the boundaries of treatment and change the transference relationship. However, I will recommend the use of yogic exercise, breathing techniques, or meditation, if their practice would be of benefit. I do refer patients to resources in the community.

My practice of yoga led to a thorough understanding of the value of healing compared with applying a fix for the symptoms, as well as an inspiration of awe in view of the extent of healing or possibility for change that is inherent in the human potential. One of the most important messages that yoga and other consciousness disciplines can teach us is the value and the chance that exist in the full experience and acceptance of the power of the present moment. As the Buddha said, when asked who he was: "I am awake." The yoking of experience and the "awake" acceptance of where "one is at" is an excellent starting point for personal growth and development in therapy.

Resources

There are a number of literature resources for physicians regarding the use of yoga in practice, including *Yoga Journal*, the largest periodical (2054 University Avenue, Berkeley, CA 94704; 510-841-9200; for subscriptions: 800-436-9642). *Light on Yoga* by B. K. S. Iyengar is a comprehensive guide to all postures and main practices of yoga with detailed lists of therapeutic practices for different physical conditions and suggested series of postures for complete practice. *Yoga Basics* by Mara Carrico is an excellent beginner's guide and introduction to yoga. *The Integral Yoga* by Sri Aurobindo, one of many volumes on his work, provides a good introduction to his ideas. *Raja Yoga* by Swami Vivekananda outlines the eight limb path and comments on the yoga sutra attributed to Patanjali. *The Heart of Yoga: Developing a Personal Practice* by T. K. V. Desikachar is an inclusive guide to the main techniques of hatha yoga and yogic philosophy, including the yoga sutra. *Light on Pranayama,* also by B. K. S. Iyengar, is a comprehensive guide to yogic breathing techniques and relaxation techniques. It contains a number of suggested courses for learning pranayama. *Be as You Are: The Teachings of Sri Ramana Maharishi,* edited by David Goodman, describes teachings on many important yogic concepts from a modern-day Indian sage. *Yoga, Immortality and Freedom* by Mircea Eliade provides a guide to yogic philosophy and cosmology. *The Yoga Tradition: Its History, Literature, Philosophy, and Practice* by Georg Feuerstein is a complete reference guide to yoga and all of its concepts and practices.

References

American Psychiatric Association: Diagnostic and Statistical Manual of Mental Disorders, 3rd Edition, Revised. Washington, DC, American Psychiatric Association, 1987

American Psychiatric Association: Diagnostic and Statistical Manual of Mental Disorders, 4th Edition. Washington, DC, American Psychiatric Association, 1994

Andrews G, Macmahon SW, Austin A, et al: Hypertension: comparison of drug and non-drug treatments. BMJ 284:1523–1526, 1982

Aurobindo S: The Integral Yoga: Sri Aurobindo's Teaching and Method of Practice. Twin Lakes, WI, Lotus Light Publications, 1993, pp 264–267

Aurobindo S: Sri Aurobindo or The Adventure of Consciousness. Satprem, Pondicherry, India, Sri Aurobindo Ashram, 1995

Berger BG, Owen DR: Mood alterations with yoga and swimming: aerobic exercise may not be necessary. Perceptual & Motor Skills 75(3 Pt 2):1331–1343, 1992

Blavatsky HP: Isis Unveiled (1877). London, England, Theosophical University Press, 1988

Blavatsky HP: The Secret Doctrine: A Synthesis of Science, Religion, and Philosophy (1888). London, England, Theosophical University Press, 1989

Carrico M: Yoga Basics. New York, Henry Holt and Company, 1997, pp 4–6, 10–15, 31–39

Dass R: Be Here Now. Albuquerque, NM, Lama Foundation, 1971

Desikachar TKV: The Heart of Yoga: Developing a Personal Practice. Rochester, VT, Inner Traditions International, 1995

Eliade M: Yoga, Immortality, and Freedom. Princeton, NJ, Princeton University Press, 1958

Epstein M: Going to Pieces Without Falling Apart: A Buddhist Perspective on Wholeness. New York, Broadway Books, 1998

Feuerstein G: The Yoga Tradition: Its History, Literature, Philosophy, and Practice. Prescott, AZ, Hohm Press, 1998, pp 253, 320–321

Folan LM: Lilias, Yoga, and You. New York, Bantam Books, 1976

Garfinkel MS, Schumacher HR Jr, Husain A, et al: Evaluation of a yoga based regimen for treatment of osteoarthritis of the hands. J Rheumatol 21(12):2341–2343, 1994

Garfinkel MS, Singhal A, Katz WA, et al: Yoga-based intervention for carpal tunnel syndrome: a randomized trial. JAMA 280:1601–1603, 1998

Goodman D: Be As You Are: The Teachings of Sri Ramana Maharishi. London, England, Arkana, 1985

Goyeche JR, Abo Y, Ikemi Y: Asthma: the yoga perspective. Part II: Yoga therapy in the treatment of asthma. J Asthma 19(3):189-201, 1982

Hatha Yoga Pradipika (with comment by Swami Muktibodhananda Saraswati). Munger (Bihar), India, Bihar School of Yoga, 1985

Hittleman RL: Richard Hittleman's Yoga: 28-Day Exercise Plan. New York, Workman Publishing, 1969

Iyengar BKS: Light on Yoga. New York, Schocken Books, 1979

Iyenger BKS: Light on Pranayama. New York, Crossroad Publishing, 1998

Jain SC, Rai L, Valecha A, et al: Effect of yoga training on exercise tolerance in adolescents with childhood asthma. J Asthma 28:437–442, 1991

Jain SC, Uppal A, Bhatnagar SO, et al: A study of response pattern of non-insulin dependent diabetics to yoga therapy. Diabetes Res Clin Pract 19:69–74, 1993

Jois KP: Yoga Mala. New York, Patanjali Yoga, 1999

Jung CG: The Psychology of Kundalini Yoga. Princeton, NJ, Princeton University Press, 1996

Kabat-Zinn J: An outpatient program in behavioral medicine for chronic pain patients based on the practice of mindfulness meditation: theoretical considerations and preliminary results. Gen Hosp Psychiatry 4:33–47, 1982

Khanam AA, Sachdeva U, Guleria R, et al: Study of pulmonary and autonomic functions of asthma patients after yoga training. Indian J Physiol Pharmacol 40:318–324, 1996

Krishna G: The Secret of Yoga. London, England, Turnstone Books, 1972

Madanmohan, Thombre DP, Balakumar B, et al: Effect of yoga training on reaction time, respiratory endurance and muscle strength. Indian J Physiol Pharmacol 36:229–233, 1992

Miller BS: Yoga Discipline of Freedom. The Yoga Sutra Attributed to Patanjali. Berkeley, CA, University of California Press, 1996

Miller JJ, Fletcher K, Kabat-Zinn J: Three-year follow-up and clinical implications of a mindfulness-based stress reduction intervention in the treatment of anxiety disorders. Gen Hosp Psychiatry 17:192–200, 1995

Monro R, Nagarathna R, Nagendra HR: Yoga for Common Ailments: A Fireside Book. New York, Simon & Schuster, 1990

Morris K: Meditating on yogic science. Lancet 351:1038, 1998

Murthy PJ: P300 amplitude and antidepressant response to Sudarshan Kriya Yoga (SKY). J Affect Disord 50:45–48, 1998

Nagarathna S: Clinical study of yoga techniques in university students with asthma: a controlled study. Allergy Asthma Proc 19:3–9, 1998

Nagendra HR, Nagarathna R: An integrated approach of yoga therapy for bronchial asthma: a 3-54 month prospective study. J Asthma 23:123–137, 1986

Ornish DM, Gotto AM, Miller RR, et al: Effects of a vegetarian diet and selected yoga techniques in the treatment of coronary heart disease. Clin Res 27:720A, 1979

Panjwani U, Selvamurthy W, Singh SH, et al: Effect of Sahaja yoga practice on seizure control and EEG changes in patients with epilepsy. Indian J Med Res 103:165–172, 1996

Raju PS, Prasad KV, Venkata RY, et al: Influence of intensive yoga training on physiological changes in 6 adult women: a case report. J Altern Complement Med 3:291–295, 1997

Rama, Ballentine R, Ajaya: Yoga and Psychotherapy: The Evolution of Consciousness. Honesdale, PA, The Himalayan International Institute of Yoga Science and Philosophy, 1990

Schell FJ: Physiological and psychological effects of hatha-yoga exercise in healthy women. Int J Psychosom 41:46–52, 1994

Schmidt T, Wijga A, Von Zur Muhlen A, et al: Changes in cardiovascular risk factors and hormones during a three month kriya yoga training and vegetarian nutrition. Acta Physiol Scand Suppl 640:158–162, 1997

Shaffer HJ, LaSalvia TA, Stein JP: Comparing hatha yoga with dynamic group psychotherapy for enhancing methadone maintenance treatment: a randomized clinical trial. Altern Ther Health Med 3:57–66, 1997

Shannahoff-Khalsa DS, Beckett LR: Clinical case report: efficacy of yogic techniques in the treatment of obsessive compulsive disorders. Int J Neurosci 85:1–17, 1996

Sharma SK, Singh B: Yoga: A Guide to Healthy Living. New Delhi, India, Lustre Press Pvt Ltd, 1997

Shivapremananda: Yoga for Stress Relief. New York, Random House, 1997

Singh V, Wisniewski A, Britton J, et al: Effect of yoga breathing exercises (pranayama) on airway reactivity in subjects with asthma. Lancet 335:1381–1383, 1990

Stancak A Jr, Kuna M: EEG changes during forced alternate nostril breathing. Int J Psychophysiol 18:75–79, 1994

Sundar S, Agrawal SK, Singh VP, et al: Role of yoga in management of essential hypertension. Acta Cardiol 39:203–208, 1984

Vahia NS, Vinekar SL, Doongaji DR: Some ancient Indian concepts in the treatment of psychiatric disorders. Br J Psychiatry 112:1089–1096, 1966

Vahia NS, Doongaji DR, Jeste DV, et al: Psychophysiological therapy based on the concepts of Patanjali: a new approach to the treatment of neurotic and psychosomatic disorders. Am J Psychother 27:557–565, 1973

Vedanthan PK, Kesavalu LN, Murthy KC, et al: Clinical study of yoga techniques in university students with asthma: a controlled study. Allergy Asthma Proc 19:3–9, 1998

Vivekananda: Raja Yoga. New York, Ramakrishna-Vivekananda Center, 1956

Walsh R: The consciousness disciplines and the behavioral sciences: questions of comparison and assessment. Am J Psychiatry 137:663–673, 1980

Weller S: Yoga Therapy. London, England, Thorsons, 1995

Wilber K: The Spectrum of Consciousness. Wheaton, IL, Theosophical Publishing House, 1977

Wilber K: No Boundary. Los Angeles, CA, Center Press, 1979

Wilber K, Engler J, Brown DP: Transformations of Consciousness: conventional and Contemplative Perspectives on Development. Boston, MA, Shambala, 1986, pp 65–105, 120–126

Wood CJ: Mood change and perception of vitality: a comparison of the effects of relaxation, visualization and yoga. J Royal Soc Med 86:254–258, 1993

Chapter 4

Meditation and Psychotherapy

Stress, Allostasis, and Enriched Learning

Joseph Loizzo, M.D., M.Phil.

Meditation in Medicine, Neuroscience, and Psychiatry

Recently, the term *meditation* has entered neuroscience and psychiatry (Kabat-Zinn et al. 1992; Kutz et al. 1985; Linehan 1993; Snaith 1998; Varela et al. 1996). Its narrow use to designate a religious practice of contemplation has broadened to include any intentional exercise of attention (Kabat-Zinn 1982). The context for this shift is the convergence of various lines of research with the introduction of Indian methods of meditation common to traditional Asian medicine and psychology (Claxton 1986; Goleman 1977; Loizzo and Blackhall 1998; Walsh 1988). The methodical nature of Indian self-regulation techniques has contributed not only to their popularity but also to their adaptation in the new fields of mind-body medicine, cognitive neuroscience, and cognitive therapy (Benson et al. 1975; Linehan et al. 1979; Varela et al. 1996). Interest in meditation as an adjunct to dynamic therapy is also increasing (Epstein 1995; Moleno 1998). As a result, psychiatrists are being asked to evaluate research and clinical alternatives involving the use of techniques that were previously dismissed as placebo practices or as obsessive rituals (Bogart 1991; Craven 1989; Holmes 1987; Snaith 1998).

For psychiatrists, the challenge posed by rising interest in meditation is part of the larger challenge posed by alternatives to conventional medicine (Berkenwald 1998; Eisenberg et al. 1993). The clinical usefulness of meditative techniques for stress-related conditions such as heart disease was established well before the recent trend toward complementary and alternative medicine (CAM) (Benson 1977; Benson and Wallace 1972). Mind-body medicine, founded on meditation-based techniques such as the relaxation response, is more evidence-based than most alternative practices and even many conventional ones (Fugh-Berman 1996) and is routinely distinguished from CAM (Goleman and Gurin 1993). The recent National Institutes of Health (NIH) initiative to fund mind-body medical centers reflects the consensus that self-regulation techniques such as meditation are of proven value for many conditions and are vital to the future of medicine. There is increasing neuroscientific evidence that the psychobiology of stress plays a critical role in many psychiatric syndromes (Fawcett 1992; Kagan et al. 1988; Schmidt et al. 1997; M. Smith et al. 1989). This lends weight to recent clinical findings that meditation-based stress-reduction techniques are effective in a broad range of psychiatric maladies (Kabat-Zinn et al. 1992; Linehan 1993; Linehan et al. 1991, 1992; Miller et al. 1995).

In addition to being evidence-based, meditative alternatives pose a unique challenge for psychiatry because their mechanisms and effects overlap with those of conventional psychiatric methods such as hypnotherapy and psychotherapy (Gruzelier and Brow 1985; Kabat-Zinn et al. 1992; Marriott 1996; Mikulas 1981; J. Smith 1987). Although this overlap is hard to define given the preliminary state of research in both fields, certain features linking meditation and psychotherapy are emerging (Bogart 1991; Marriott 1996; D. Shapiro 1987; J. Smith 1987). Beyond their use as relaxation techniques, Indian systems of self-regulation such as Hindu yoga and Buddhist meditation pose unique challenges as alternative therapies (Claxton 1986; Kelly 1996; Walsh 1988; West 1987). Unlike modern alternatives, these Asian methods are more ambitious in nature and scope, with coherent systems of theory, practice, and education that have withstood the centuries and adapted to diverse civilizations (Goleman 1977; Thurman 1984; Walsh 1988). They challenge researchers and clinicians not just because they are more ambitious and complete than modern techniques, such as hypnosis or psychoanalysis, but also because, like hypnosis and psychoanalysis, they involve systems of theory and practice that strike many as arbitrary and unscientific (Bogart 1991; Carrington 1978; Holmes 1987).

Alternative medical research offers three approaches to the problem: 1) If meditative practices are reducible to the placebo effect, how do we prove this without studying them in their entirety (Holmes 1987)? 2) If meditative practices are effective techniques embedded in prescientific systems, how do we distill their active ingredients (Benson et al. 1975; Carrington 1987)? 3) If Asian systems of meditation involve something akin to a scientific psychology and empirical therapeutics, how do we learn what they have to offer as coherent systems to modern psychiatry (Loizzo and Blackhall 1998)? In this chapter I explore the third approach, weighing the strongest arguments and evidence supporting the potential contribution that the world's meditation traditions can make in modern psychiatry against the conceptual and methodologic challenges (Bradwejn et al. 1985; Delmonte 1987; D. Shapiro 1987; Walsh 1996). This requires a review of the current state of meditation research and clinical application and demands a perspective and a method that diverge in ways from the usual review format. Any useful introduction to this field requires a cross-cultural perspective as well as correlating preliminary data with findings from related fields. Reference to traditional concepts, key Sanskrit technical terms (see Table 4–1), and data from a handful of basic research fields makes for unusual psychiatric reading but is essential given the preliminary state of current knowledge (Walsh 1996).

From Meditation to Psychotherapy: The Bridge of Hypnotic Learning

In this chapter, I employ a cross-cultural comparative framework based on learning models of meditation, hypnosis, and psychotherapy. First, however, I must provide some historical perspective.

Early Meditation Research

Although meditation research began in the field with the first portable electroencephalograms (EEGs) (Anand et al. 1961; Bagchi and Wegner 1957; Das and Gastaut 1955; Kasamatsu et al.

Table 4–1. Key Sanskrit terms and English equivalents

English term and synonyms	Sanskrit term and equivalents
action	*karma*
addictive behavior	*kliṣṭa-karma*
addictive responses or addictions	*kleśa*
alertness	*samprajanya*
analytic insight	*vipaśyana*, Pāli *vipassana*
attention	*manaskāra*
attentional alteration or contemplation	*dhyāna*
attentional absorption or trance	*samāpatti*
body, matter, somatic system	*śarīra, rūpa, rūpa-skandha*
central neural pathways and complexes	*suṣumṇa-nadī-chakra*
concentrative quiescence	*śamatha*
cognition, cognitive system	*jñāna, saṃjñā, saṃjñā-skandha*
compassion or empathy	*karuṇā*
compulsive behavior	*upādana-karma*
concentration	*samādhi*
concentrative quiescence	*śamatha*
consciousness, consciousness system	*vijñāna, vijñāna-skandha*
construction, construct	*vikalpana, vikalpa*
contemplation	*dhyāna*
creative imagery or creation stage	*utpatti-krama*
defensive reactivity or self-protective habit	*ātmagrahabandha*
devotional practices, devotional service	*bhakti-sevā*
egocentric instinct or self-protective instinct	*ātmagrahavāsanā*
emotion, emotional system	*saṃskāra, saṃskāra-skandha*
empathy or compassion	*karuṇā*
euphoria-mediated insight	*abheda-sukha-śūnya-jñāna*
euphoric openness or undivided bliss-void	*abedha-sukha-śūnya*
exclusive, narrow, or single-pointed concentration	*ekagraha-samādhi*
focus	*anuvṛtti*

Table 4–1. Key Sanskrit terms and English equivalents *(continued)*

English term and synonyms	Sanskrit term and equivalents
freedom	*vimokṣa*
giving and taking	Tibetan *gtong-len*
great perfection	*mahāniṣpanna*, Tibetan *rdzogs-chen*
great seal or universal seal meditation	*mahāmūdra*
guide or expert guide	*kalayānamitra*
higher education or reeducation	*adhisikṣya*
instinctive or unconscious responses	*svabhāvavikalpa*
inclusive, open or spacious equipoise	*akāśopama-samahita*
individual vehicle	*hinayāna*, Pāli *Theravada*
insight or wisdom	*prajñā*
cognitive or intellectually acquired insight	*śruta-mayī-prajñā*
affective or reflectively acquired insight	*cinta-mayī-prajñā*
behavioral or meditatively acquired insight	*bhāvanā-mayī-prajñā*
intention	*cetana*
intuitive clarity or lucid insight	*prabhāsvara-jñāna*
intuitive realization or perfection stage	*niṣpanna-krama*
imagery-mediated insight or indivisible appearance-voidness insight	*abheda-pratibha-śūnyatá-jñāna*
imaginative schema or visualized environment	*maṇḍala*
kindling, inner fire, or psychic heat	*caṇḍali*, Tibetan *gTum-mo*
loving-kindness or love	*maitrī*, Pāli *metta*
lucid insight or intuitive clarity	*prabhāsvara-jñāna*
meditation	*bhāvanā, dhyāna*
mentor	*gūru*
mind	*citta, manas*
mind-body process or integration process	*yoga-tantra*
mindfulness	*smṛti*, Pāli *sati*
mind-training or mind-reform	*blo-byong*
mnemonic formula	*mantra, dhāraṇī*
motivation	*chandana*

Table 4–1. Key Sanskrit terms and English equivalents *(continued)*

English term and synonyms	Sanskrit term and equivalents
neural complex	*cakra*
neural energy	*prāṇa*
neural pathway	*nadī*
neurotransmitter, modulator, or secretion	*bindu*
noble truths	*āryasatya*
truth of suffering	*duḥkhā-satya*
truth of reinforcement or origin	*samudaya-satya*
truth of extinction	*nirvāṇa-satya*
truth of the path	*mārga-satya*
nonconceptual concentration	*nirvikalpasamādhi*
nondualistic insight	*advaityajñāna*
nonrelational or intrinsic identity	*svalakṣaṇa*
nonrelational or intrinsic reality	*svabhāva*
openness or voidness	*śūnyatā*
optimal mind-body process or unexcelled integration process	*anuttarayogatantra*
orgasmic euphoria or innate bliss	*sahaja-sukha*
passion practice	*rāga-dharma*
perception	*sparśa, pratyakṣa*
plasticity, pliancy, or fluency	*praśrabdhi*
process vehicle	*tantrayāna*
prosocial emotions or boundless attitudes	*apramāṇa-dhyāna*
pure or real bliss consciousness	*sat-cit-ānanda*
quiescence meditation	*śamatha-bhāvanā*
reeducation or higher education	*adhisikṣya*
reeducation in insight or wisdom	*prajñā-adhisikṣya*
reeducation in mindset or meditation	*samādhi-adhisikṣya*
reeducation in lifestyle or ethics	*śilā-adhisikṣya*
relativity or conditioned development	*idampratyāyatā, pratītyasamutpāda*
reliance	*pratisāraṇa*
resistance or obscuration	*āvaraṇa*
cognitive resistance	*jñeyāvaraṇa*

Table 4–1. Key Sanskrit terms and English equivalents *(continued)*

English term and synonyms	Sanskrit term and equivalents
affective resistance	*kleśāvaraṇa*
sensation, sensory system	*vedanā, vedanā-skandha*
sexual arousal	*śṛngārānurāgana*
single vehicle	*ekayāna*
social field	*sattvaksetra*
social or universal vehicle	*mahāyāna*
state of mind, state of consciousness	*manasāyatana, vijñānasthiti*
subconscious mind	*ālayavijñāna*
sympathy	*sahṛdaya*
teacher	*śāstṛ*
therapeutic technique or liberative art	*upāya-kauśalya*
therapeutic vehicle or liberative method	*yāna*
individual vehicle	*hinayāna*, Pāli *Theravada*
social or universal vehicle	*mahāyāna*
process, creative or diamond vehicle	*tantrayāna, mantrayāna, vajrayāna*
transcendent insight	*prajñāpāramitā*
translucency or clear light	*prabhāsvara*
unconditional empathy or compassion	*anupalambha-karuṇā*
virtual body or illusion body	*māyadeha*
visualized environment or imaginative schema	*maṇḍala*
voidness or openness	*śūnyatā*

1957), Western conceptions about Indian meditation were shaped by the introduction of transcendental meditation (TM), a scientifically framed, tradition-based technique that consists of adopting certain postures (from hatha yoga) while focusing on a mnemonic formula (*mantra*) recited subvocally. Research showed that the technique of sustaining single-pointed concentration on a chosen stimulus induced a more or less profound hypometabolic, hyperattentive state (R. Wallace et al. 1971). In advanced practitioners, it often yielded a euphoric, nonconceptual absorption described as "pure consciousness" (Banquet 1973). Early conceptions of meditation as a more or less profound but unitary state of relaxed alertness were reinforced when Herbert Benson developed a TM-based method of inducing a relaxation response that could reduce stress reactivity and psychophysiologic activation (Beary and Benson 1974; Benson et al. 1975). Initial findings that this method worked for managing stress, hypertension, and other cardiac disorders were extended to a range of problems from addiction to anxiety (Beary and Benson 1974; Benson and Wallace 1971, 1972; Benson et al. 1975, 1978), laying the foundations for mind-body medicine. Researchers observed that meditative and hypnotic subjects shared certain predisposing variables and that EEG studies of TM and hypnosis showed common state markers (Bushell 1998). This finding led to comparisons of the techniques and a conception of meditation as a trance that helps control automatic processes by attentional alterations that heighten susceptibility to autosuggestion (Delmonte 1981, 1984c; Gruzelier and Brow 1985; Heide et al. 1980; Van Nuys 1973). Variations in the depth of the meditative state were explained (as in hypnosis) by predisposition and skill variables that made the state more or less effective in facilitating conscious self-regulation and long-term change. Because this conception accurately describes the early stages of concentrative meditation (*samadhi* or *shamatha*) (e.g., Banquet's [1973] TM stages 1 and 2), it is still widely accepted (Snaith 1998).

Mindfulness

Later understanding advanced in two ways. Exploration of the variety of Asian meditative practices revealed their experiential and biological diversity (Goleman 1977; West 1987), and further studies of concentrative meditation helped differentiate these practices from normal rest, sleep, and hypnosis (Davidson and Goleman 1977; Infante et al. 1998; Jevning et al. 1992, 1996). Key to exploring the variety of meditative practices was the introduction of analytic insight meditation, commonly called *mindfulness* (Kabat-Zinn 1990). Basic mindfulness meditation (*smrti* or *sati* in the Pali dialect) involves trying to sustain attention from moment to moment on a chosen focus in the body or mind. Typically, the first focus is the breath, which serves both as the paradigm for the practice of deautomatizing mind-body processes (Deikman 1966) and as the induction vehicle for the relaxed alert state on which advanced practice depends (Morse et al. 1984). Although basic mindfulness practice and concentrative meditation are indistinguishable at early stages (Brown 1977; A. Wallace 1999), mindfulness diverges in its advanced stages; it opens the focus of attention to admit whatever enters experience while using relaxed alertness to maintain an observational stance of impartial attention. This impartial attention investigates whatever appears without the bias of habitual judgments or emotional reactivity. This final discipline of mindfulness is traditionally defined as analytic insight meditation (*vipasyana* or *vipassana* in Pali), in which discursive intellect is used before, during, and after meditation sessions as part of a threefold education aimed at personal freedom and change (Mikulas 1978, 1981). The explosion of interest in mindfulness was fueled by evidence that it enhances learning-related attentional variables such as perceptual discrimination (Brown et al. 1984) while promoting the development of positive psychobiologic traits such as sense of coherence and stress-hardiness (Davidson and Goleman 1977; Easterlin and Cardena 1998; Kabat-Zinn et al. 1997). Growing understanding of mindfulness and analytic insight meditation helped researchers explain inconsistent findings from meditation studies using practitioners from different traditions (Delmonte 1984a). New frameworks of meditative experience based on classical Indian mindfulness literature were developed (Goleman 1977) to map the relations between various Indian practices and to locate Jewish, Christian, Islamic, Central Asian, and East Asian Buddhist practices.

The Learning Model

As the varieties of meditation were being categorized and compared, further research on TM and the most advanced practices of Hindu and Buddhist tantric yoga was highlighting the biological distinctiveness and self-regulatory scope of meditative states (Benson et al. 1982; Heller et al. 1987; Jevning et al. 1992). From the finding that the state-trait decreases in stress reactivity in TM involved alterations not only in response set but also in stimulus set, researchers concluded that the mechanisms and effects of meditation were more profound than those of hypnosis and involved learning and neural plasticity (Davidson and Goleman 1977; Gruzelier and Brow 1985; Mikulas 1981). This learning model gained support from clinical studies suggesting that mindfulness was effective in pain, anxiety, and borderline personality disorder because it enhanced learning by increasing attentional competence (Kabat-Zinn 1982; Kabat-Zinn et al. 1992; Linehan 1993). This shift in meditation models was congruent with developments in hypnosis research that suggested hypnotherapy worked by heightening attention and enhancing problem solving and learning (Bushell 1998; DePascalis and Penna 1990; Sabourin et al. 1990). The consensus that meditation and hypnosis are similar and are both better explained as learning, rather than as suggestion, offers a bridge from meditation to psychotherapy, for example, Freud's "waking-state hypnosis"(Marriott 1996). Before crossing this bridge, however, the new learning models of meditation must be grounded cross-culturally in a comparative framework of meditation.

Learning models of meditation may challenge common conceptions, but classical Indian models treat meditative self-regulation as part of a path of higher learning whose three tracks involve cognitive, affective, and behavioral reeducation (*adhisiksya*). Reeducation is viewed as a continuing process, with three developmental phases aimed at progressive insight (*prajna*) based on intellectual, reflective, and meditative learning. In addition to clarifying traditional learning models, recent scholarship also offers more complete maps of meditation. Goleman's (1977) fifth-century source omits later developments, including the more advanced mind-body process (*yoga tantra*) techniques that would set the gold standard for effectiveness (Benson et al. 1990; Heller et al. 1987; Isayeva 1995; Thurman 1998). The framework I adapt is based on Indo-Tibetan Buddhist sources ranging from Atisha (982–1054) to Tsong Khapa (1493–1517) (Thurman 1984, 1998). One of the advantages of this framework is that it was developed in dialogue with the Hindu tradition and may be easily coordinated with frameworks based on the synthesis of Abhinavagupta (c. 1000), such as that of Sri Aurobindo (Isayeva 1995).

Given this framework of meditation, we can cross the bridge from hypnotherapy to learning models in psychotherapy. Appreciation of the constructive role played by internal variables in learning has led to the modified behavioral model of cognitive-behavioral therapy (CBT) (Beck et al. 1979) and to related moves to integrate analytic and learning models of dynamic therapy (Luborsky 1984). Greater dialogue with neurobiology (Rieser 1984) has made psychotherapy researchers aware that learning plays a formative role in the development of brain structure and function and that its substrate, neural plasticity, is a pervasive and continuous property of neural systems rather than the exception to a rule of genetically determined "hard-wiring" (Kandel and Schwartz 1991). The biology of learning has been invoked as a final common pathway in the mechanisms of action of the major classes of psychopharmacologic agents (Hyman and Nestler 1996) and has been cited as the foundation for a new scientific framework for psychiatry (Kandel 1999). Combining this framework with developments in mind-body medicine and neuroscience will complete the comparative learning model and help schematize the discussion to follow.

From Trauma to Enrichment: Stress, Learning, and the Brain

Stress

In recent years, research on the mechanisms and effects of stress has opened a new window on the pathogenesis of mental illness (Fawcett 1992; Kagan et al. 1988; Schmidt et al. 1997; M. Smith et al. 1989). The triphasic sequence of events observed in the general stress response—1) fear-based cognition, 2) aversive effect, and 3) hypothalamic-pituitary-adrenal (HPA) activation leading to decreased neurogenesis, long-term degradation of neural tissue, and decreased cortical volume—is also at work in the genesis of psychologic trauma, anxiety, and mood disorders (Bremner et al. 1995; Carroll 1991; Coplan et al. 1996; Darnell et al. 1994; Drevets et al. 1992; Sheline et al. 1996; Starkman et al. 1993; Yehuda 1997). Selective serotonin reuptake inhibitors (SSRIs) are now thought to reverse the degradation process and promote neural plasticity by increasing nerve growth factors in the hippocampus and prefrontal cortex (Haddjeri et al. 1998), supporting learning models of depression as a neural plasticity disorder. The allostasis model from mind-body medical research promises to be helpful in the assessment of the pathologic effects of uncontrollable stress:

> Allostasis means achieving stability through change, and it refers in part to the process of increasing sympathetic and hypothalamic pituitary adrenal activity to promote adaptation and to reestablish homeostasis. Allostasis also highlights our ability to anticipate, adapt or cope with impending future events . . . when allostatic systems remain active they can cause wear and tear on tissues and accelerate pathophysiology—a phenomenon we have called allostatic load. . . . There are three types of allostatic load: 1) frequent overstimulation by frequent stress, resulting in excessive hormone exposure, 2) failure to turn off allostatic responses when they are not needed or inability to habituate to the same stressor, both of which result in overexposure to stress hormones, 3) inability to turn on allostatic responses when needed, in which case other systems (e.g. inflammatory cytokines) become hyperactive and produce other types of wear and tear. (Shulkin et al. 1998, p. 220)

In this and prior articles, Shulkin et al. (1994) proposed a general mechanism for allostatic load based on tonically increased fear due to stress-conditioned amygdalar hyperactivity. They asserted that a broad range of psychiatric disorders—from anxiety, posttraumatic stress disorder (PTSD), addictions, and depression to Alzheimer's disease and schizophrenia—reflects a spectrum of psychopathology caused or accelerated by wear and tear due to allostatic load. The continuum of types 1, 2, and 3 allostatic load could account for the nonspecificity of psychiatric symptoms such as negative anticipation, aversive reactivity, and learned helplessness. This model also highlights the constructive role of the individual in biobehavioral responses as well as the exorbitant hidden cost to the mind and brain of the failure to relearn the conditioned fear responses that maintain allostatic load. Pinpointing defensive reactivity as a prime risk factor and a common pathway to mental disorders helps to align psychiatric nosology with mind-body medical findings that trace the pervasive pathologic effects of disease-prone behaviors to the defensive psychologic traits of self-involvement, fearful attachment, and hostility (Scherwitz et al. 1986; Williams 1989).

Learning

Although psychiatric researchers have recognized the therapeutic implications of findings that cortisol-mediated hippocampal damage can be reversed by decreasing cortisol levels (Seeman et al. 1997), they have interpreted those implications narrowly as confirming the plasticity model of SSRI action and the need for more plasticity agents. Researchers in geriatrics and rehabilitation have explored the effectiveness of cognitive-affective-behavioral strategies for enhancing plasticity, neurogenesis, memory, and learning (Carney et al. 1999; Farmer and Clippard 1994; Sohlberg and Mateer 1989; Swaab 1991). The rationale for these strategies comes from animal studies of the effects of enriched environments on learning (Bushell 1998; Rosensweig and Bennett 1996; Ryff and Singer 1998; Swaab 1991). Four decades of research on the hypothesis of use-induced plasticity of the nervous system have shown that training or enriched experience induces dramatic changes in the cerebral cortex of rats and other animals. Training or enriched experience altered neurochemistry, increased cortical weight and thickness, enhanced size of synaptic contacts and number of dendritic spines and branchings, and improved performance on tests of learning, and did so more or less independently of age (Rosensweig and Bennett 1996). The data are remarkable both qualitatively and quantitatively, showing increases in some variables of up to 10%–25% with as little exposure as 40 minutes per day (Ferchmin and Ertovic 1989; Greenough and Volkmar 1973; Ng and Gibbs 1991). Extension to humans is supported by findings that adults who continue learning retain higher brain size and capacity (Schaie 1994; Shimamura et al. 1995). Equally dramatic is the inverse effect of impoverishment (Wiesel and Hubel 1965). How do we explain the discrepant effects of stressful versus enriched environments, that is, "wear and tear" versus "use it or lose it"? The current consensus is that use-dependent plasticity is the rule and stress-induced atrophy the exception (Rosensweig and Bennett 1996; Ryff and Singer 1998; Swaab 1991).

Table 4–2. Stages of integrated concentrative and analytic meditation

Concentration	Skills	Motivation	Insight
Individual phase	**Low arousal**	**Exclusive attention**	**Cognitive learning**
Focus	Learning	Relief	Discursive
Steady focus	Reflection	Renunciation	Analytic
Repeated focus	Mindfulness	Impartiality	Holistic
Increased focus	Mindfulness	Equanimity	Perceptual
Social phase	**Low arousal**	**Inclusive attention**	**Affective learning**
Discipline	Alertness	Concern	Intuitive
Calm	Alertness	Compassion	Imaginative
Quiescence	Effort	Care	Visceral
Process phase	**High arousal**	**Integrative attention**	**Behavioral learning**
One-pointedness	Effort	Commitment	Euphoric
Equipoise	Plasticity	Altruism	Orgasmic

Source. Thurman 1984.

Effects on the Brain

Given a cognitive-affective-behavioral learning model, the negative effects of stress and the positive effects of enrichment on the brain are consistent with the reciprocal inhibition of aversive and reward learning systems hypothesized by researchers for decades (Block 1977; Bushell 1998; Doidge 1990; Heath 1963; MacLean 1959). Although the effects of stress are mediated by fear-based aversive arousal of amygdala-maintained (aminergic) defensive responses, the effects of enrichment are thought to be mediated by trust-based euphoric arousal and disarming (endorphinergic-oxytocinergic) sexual-nurturant responses maintained by septal-hippocampal reward circuitry, periorbital cortex, and the bed nucleus of the stria terminalis (Bushell 1998; Panksepp 1998). In the following sections, I incorporate models of allostatic load and environmental enrichment into the comparative learning framework I developed above in order to review the mechanisms of meditation.

Meditation and Psychotherapy: Two Methods of Enriched Learning

The Indo-Tibetan framework of meditative practices divides the path of insight into three progressive developmental phases and prescribes for each a distinct therapeutic technique or vehicle (Table 4–2). Fundamental is the individual vehicle (*hinayana*), which is aimed at developing the insight required for freedom from compulsive behavior (*karma*) and addictive responses (*klesha*). It prescribes a technique of impartial observation known as mindfulness or insight meditation, practiced with an attitude of renunciation, especially within the South Asian tradition. Intermediate is the social vehicle (*mahayana*), aimed at developing self-transcendent insight and unconditional empathy. It prescribes analytic insight integrated with concentrative quiescence and practiced with an attitude of universal compassion, especially in Central and East Asian traditions. Finally, the process vehicle (*tantrayana*) aims at a visceral insight called *translucency* that is integrated with a virtual body of euphoric compassion. It prescribes techniques of intuitive self-analysis within visualized environments (*manda-la*) that are perfected by the experience of orgasmic openness, and is practiced with an attitude of euphoric compassion, especially in the Tibetan tradition. This simple schema is more friendly than prior maps to the mind-body process techniques of advanced Hindu yoga practices (Patanjali stages 5–8) such as raja yoga (TM stage 3/TM-Sidhi), and also has the advantage that its developmental phases permit cross-cultural and structural-functional comparisons. Specifically, individual practices are comparable with classical analytic and cognitive therapies; social practices are comparable with object-relations approaches and interpersonal and group therapies; and process practices are comparable with Jungian and Reichian analysis, hypnotherapy, and intimacy work. Structurally and functionally, the three developmental phases may be conceptualized as facilitating relearning and plasticity at the neocortical, limbic, and subcortical levels (i.e., in encoding, registration, and commitment phases supporting short-, intermediate-, and long-term memory) in line with MacLean's (1959) comparative biological "triune brain" version of Freud's structural model (see Panksepp's revision [1998]).

Individual Meditative Practices

The first body of evidence to consider in examining this schematic framework pertains to mindfulness meditation and its relation to free association and cognitive therapy. Although mindfulness practice usually begins by focusing attention on the breath, its final application involves maintaining a nonreactive observational stance of open, impartial attention toward whatever enters the field of awareness. The effectiveness of mindfulness in treating anxiety disorders and chronic pain is thought to reflect its general health benefits, including decreased anxiety and increased stress-hardiness, rather than a disease-specific mechanism (Kabat-Zinn 1982). This concept agrees with the four noble truths (aryasatya) framework of individual self-healing, in which self-imposed suffering is approached generally, as the product of misguided behavior whose reinforcement must be understood before its extinction (nirvana) can be realized by a path of cognitive-affective-behavioral reeducation (Claxton 1987; Govinda 1974). The mechanism postulated for the effects of mindfulness involves a state of relaxed alertness in which somatic deactivation fosters an observational stance of heightened attention, open to normally automatic processes yet uncoupled from affective-behavioral reactivity (Kabat-Zinn et al. 1992). The general benefits of mindfulness are explained by the role heightened attention plays as the final common pathway and rate-limiting step in cognitive-behavioral learning (Goleman 1977; Kabat-Zinn 1982).

Discussion of the mechanism of meditation has focused on three questions pertinent to mindfulness: 1) the relation of meditative states to rest, 2) whether the attentional shift in meditation is toward opening or narrowing, and 3) the relation of this shift to cerebral laterality. Although the physiology of many common meditative practices resembles relaxed alertness from rest to the onset of stage 1 sleep, reported differences in metabolism and consciousness are regarded as sufficient to mark meditative states as psychobiologically discrete (Delmonte 1984c, 1985, 1987; Jevning et al. 1992; R. Wallace et al. 1971; Walsh 1996). EEG findings relevant to basic mindfulness practice—decreased alpha frequency and increased alpha amplitude and coherence with frontal spread—are indistinguishable from drowsiness, although nonmeditators are generally unable to stop the progression of drowsiness into stage 1 sleep, whereas meditators routinely can (Fenwick 1987). In general, debate over whether meditation is more calming than rest reflects the common misperception that the aim of meditation is relaxation. Like free association, mindfulness may be best understood as a cultivated state in which the normal progression from waking to sleep onset is stopped and exploited for deautomatizing insight and long-term change rather than as a fourth state of consciousness (Delmonte 1995; Holmes 1987).

The question of attentional alterations is raised by the contrasting modes of attention found in Hindu yoga versus Zen meditation. Using the finding that resting alpha is normally blocked by stimulation as a measure of responsiveness, early field studies of Indian yogins reported that blocking was absent, suggesting nonresponsiveness (Bagchi and Wegner 1957; Das and Gastaut 1955), whereas similar studies of Zen meditators showed that blocking not only was present but did not habituate as usual, suggesting enhanced responsiveness (Kasamatsu and Harai 1966). Eventually, these data were taken as confirming the distinctive attentional alterations in two main types of meditation: 1) concentrative meditation aimed at single-pointed focus yields exclusive heightened attention, and 2) mindfulness meditation aimed at impartial focus yields inclusive heightened attention (Davidson 1976). Although subsequent studies on TM practitioners showed inconsistent results, the consensus that these discrepant findings are the result of different voluntary alterations of attention still stands and is supported by evoked potential studies (Baumgartner and Epstein 1982; Fenwick 1987; Ikemi 1988). The attentional alterations in meditation seem to involve nonspecific mechanisms for altering cortical responsiveness that cannot fully distinguish meditation from other methods of deautomatization, such as yoga, imagery, and qi gong (Fenwick 1987; Ikemi 1988; Karawatt 1991; Liu et al. 1990).

Some researchers have proposed that the essential mechanism of meditation is a shift in cerebral dominance from the left to right hemisphere (Fenwick 1987). Early debate focused on whether the shift was due to right hemisphere activation (Davidson 1976; Ornstein 1972) or left hemisphere deactivation (Erlichman and Weiner 1980; Prince 1978). The current consensus supports varying degrees of right hemisphere activation as a mechanism in early stages and bihemispheric deactivation in more advanced stages (Earle 1984; Fenwick 1987; Liu et al. 1990). Although much of the reasoning behind this debate is based on the overgeneralization (from TM) that suppression of thought and repetition of mnemonic formulas are essential to meditation, some degree of right hemisphere activation appears in mindfulness despite its use of left hemisphere activating analysis and lack of right hemisphere activating repetition. Tachistoscopic studies of mindfulness show enhanced perceptual discrimination indicating right hemispheric activation (Brown et al. 1984). Increased meditative access to right hemisphere–stored negative emotions has also been cited by proponents of right hemisphere activation (Davidson et al. 1976) and is typically reported in mindfulness (Delmonte 1989, 1995; Miller 1993).

Right hemisphere activation and access to negative emotion have also been invoked in several biological models of psycho-

analysis (Delmonte 1989, 1995; Kissen 1986; Reiser 1984). Antici-
pating Freud, traditional descriptions of mindfulness or insight
meditation insist that attention, even single-pointed, nonconceptual concentration, is not an end in itself but a means to support
the integration of mind-body systems with analytic insight
through autointerpretation (Gimello 1978). The insistence that analytic insight is essential to mindfulness would favor the model
of balanced hemispheric dominance; enhanced cortical task spec-
ificity and integration would thus be the mechanism of both basic
mindfulness practice and access to more profound meditative self-
analysis. Support for such an integrated-systems model is found
in state theories of hypnosis (Gruzelier and Brow 1985), in studies
of hemispheric integration in meditative breathing (Jella and
Shannahoff-Khalsa 1993; Naveen et al. 1997; Persinger 1993; Stancak and Kuna 1994), and in brain imaging studies of meditation
(Herzog et al. 1991).

Mindfulness reflects the integrated effect of the manipulation
of relaxed alertness, the coherence of restful corticothalamic alpha
activation, and the balance in hemispheric dominance. Such individual self-healing practices allow the analytic hemisphere to
recruit the entire neocortical-thalamic-reticular axis (neomamma-
lian brain) for cognitively enriched learning (encoding) without
the automatic defensive appraisals that maintain cognitive-per-
ceptual allostatic load (Anand et al. 1961; Banquet 1973; Emavardhana and Tori 1997; Gellhorn and Kiely 1972; Jevning et al. 1992;
Rubin 1985).

Social Meditative Practices

Social meditative practices prescribe the most extensive use of discursive analytic insight and prosocial affective techniques. Their
analysis seems calculated to remedy any allostatic load caused by
defensive responses to psychosocial stressors. The idea is to analyze concepts and perceptions of self as supposedly fixed, or
based on some nonrelational identity or reality. This analysis
helps develop insight of the sheer relativity of self and world,
negatively defined as the voidness of such reified self-constructs.
Hindu forms of analysis focus on nondualistic insight and sym-
pathy. The common aim is to overcome conscious and uncon-

scious resistance to the self-transcendent insight and empathy on which social health depends.

The effects and mechanisms of social practices have been explored in a classic study of Zen priests (Kasamatsu and Harai 1966). Zen integrates concentrative and analytic techniques as basic training for Zazen meditation, which is typical of such practices. Zazen meditators use discursive reason or poetic formulas (*koans*) to analyze dualistic self-concepts and reactive emotions and to cultivate nondualistic insight and impartial empathy toward the world. This study of Zazen has been influential because of its methodology and significant findings. After an initial stage of alpha change, as in mindfulness and TM stage 1 and 2, the tracings of some priests showed rhythmic trains of theta waves (6–7 Hz) not seen in sleep. There was a direct correlation between these trains of theta waves and years of meditative experience. A more direct correlation was found between the theta trains and the Zen master's rating of priests as low, middle, or high in advancement. Theta trains were blocked by a sensory stimulus, and this blocking did not show habituation as in normal sleep or waking. The latter finding was interpreted as supporting the meditators' reports that they experienced the world more immediately than in normal waking but without habitual dualism or reactivity.

Hypnosis research supports this interpretation, linking enhanced theta in the 5.5–7.5 Hz range with improvements in problem-solving, perceptual processing, and cognitive and experimental task performance as well as with increased temporal blood flow (Crawford et al. 1989; Sabourin et al. 1990; Schacter 1977). Unlike the theta rhythm found in rest and drowsiness, this theta rhythm is associated with class II inhibition and is correlated with absorptive and selective attentional skills, imagery-mediated mentation, and efficient and attentive performance (Barr et al. 1995; Sabourin et al. 1990). The EEG findings, combined with the heightened sense of clarity, equanimity, and empathic relatedness reported by the priests, support the suggestion that such practices involve activating and/or integrating the temporal lobes with the frontolimbic reward system mediated by septal-hippocampal circuitry (Fenwick 1987; Mandell 1979). One case study of ecstatic seizures showed rhythmic 6- to 8-Hz theta waves during euphoric experience (Ciringotta et al. 1980). This finding suggests the possibility that the long-term changes the Zen master rated may be explained by a kindling mechanism similar to that used to explain changes in interictal personality in temporal lobe epilepsy (TLE) (Bushell 1998; Persinger 1993).

Some researchers reject kindling models of long-term meditative change, arguing that they pathologize meditation and ignore its therapeutic effects (Orme-Johnson 1995). Yet psychiatric research suggests that the interictal changes seen in euphoric TLE are so clearly adaptive that this subgroup should not be considered pathologic (Bear et al. 1985; Carroll 1991; Doidge 1990; Fieve 1997). The case would be even stronger for meditators who consciously self-regulate kindling for therapeutic benefit and adaptive change (Bushell 1998). In this view, social meditation exploits the feed-forward facilitation and long-lasting afterdischarge typical of septal-hippocampal circuitry (Adey et al. 1962; Spencer and Kandel 1961) in order to self-induce long-term potentiation (presumably by selective self-stimulation of hypothalamic reward circuits) (Slawinska and Kasicki 1995), thereby fostering the long-term learning of prosocial insights and emotions.

Through deepening relaxed alertness and hemispheric integration into the limbic system, social meditation practices appear to selectively recruit the prosocial reward mode of the frontolimbic-hypothalamic axis (the paleomammalian brain). This results in effectively enriched learning (registration) by activating septal-hippocampal inhibition of the defensive (amygdaloid) reactivity that maintains perceptual-affective allostatic load (Davidson 1976; Mandell 1979; Persinger 1984, 1993).

Process Meditative Practices

Finally, process practices combine mantra recitation, visualization, and breath-control techniques to yield deeper forms of restful alertness as well as lucid forms of rapid eye movement (REM) and non-REM sleep, sexual intercourse, and near-death experience. These lucid altered states are used to analyze defensive self-image, affect, and action and to integrate automatic mind-body processes with a creative process of intuitive clarity and euphoric openness, or pure bliss consciousness. Research on these practices began when one of the first field studies contradicted prior concepts of meditation as relaxation (Das and Gastaut 1955). Autonomic and EEG markers of increased arousal were observed during the most profound meditations of the most experienced subjects. These findings were replicated in subsequent studies of various process techniques (Bagchi and Wegner 1957; Banquet 1973; Benson et al. 1982, 1990; Corby et al. 1978). Arousal markers, such as increased heart rate, cerebral blood flow, and galvanic skin response (GSR) and stable, high-frequency beta (20–40 Hz) in meditating EEG were all the more intriguing because they were linked with paradoxical findings of peripheral deactivation, such as profound reductions in basal metabolism (40%–64%) (Benson et al. 1982, 1990; Heller et al. 1987; Infante et al. 1998; Jevning et al. 1992; Narayan et al. 1990).

Although repetition of mnemonic formulas has often been cited in models of meditation as right hemisphere–dominated waking, it is a distinctive process technique used to reinforce imaginative schemas (*mandalas*) that induce paradoxical arousal states more comparable with the "heart-brain preparation" seen in REM sleep than with the relaxed alertness found in mindfulness, Zazen, or stages 1, 2, and 4 TM (Jevning et al. 1992). The traditions view these lucid, high-arousal states and their imagery-meditated analysis as means of accessing deeper states of euphoric arousal, linked on their map of conscious self-regulation with the primary core neural pathways, complexes, energies, and transmitters (*nadi, chakra, prana, bindu*) that support appetites, consciousness, and vital functions, including plasticity (*prashrabdhi*). A study of Tibetan optimal mind-body process (*anuttara yoga tantra*) meditators who had progressed beyond the creative imagery stage to the bliss-meditated self-analysis of the intuitive realization stage documented their ability to self-regulate body temperature and metabolism. This self-regulation was taken as a gross measure of progress in the basic realization-stage euphoric technique of kindling (*candali* or *gTum-mo* in Tibetan). The most advanced practitioner was the one found to have the paradoxical arousal pattern of reduced metabolism with high-frequency beta (Benson et al. 1982, 1990).

The imagery used to induce kindling belongs to a passion practice in which virtual or real intercourse yields orgasmic bliss. This bliss is used to support lucid euphoric analysis and disarm defensive responses. Passion practice may account for reports of virtuoso process practitioners whose meditating EEGs show global activation comparable with that correlated with orgasmic experience during direct stimulation of reward circuitry in the human brain (Funderburk 1977; Green et al. 1970; Heath 1963). Current imagery research shows that structured imagery is a reliable method of inducing specific effects, and that vivid mental imagery acts as a centrally generated sensory stimulus that can be regulated to yield precise control over a wide range of automatic processes (Bushell 1998; Kosslyn 1994; Kunzendorf and Sheikh 1990). As for the traditional model of disarming defensive responses, researchers cite replicated studies of process virtuosos enduring air-tight burial for days at a time (Anand et al. 1961; Heller et al. 1987) or voluntarily suspending respiration and heartbeat (Farrow and Herbert 1982; Funderburk 1977). Direct and indirect support for traditional claims of lucid REM or slow-wave sleep may be found in recent studies of lucid deep sleep, lucid dreaming, and anesthetic recall (Gackenbach 1992; Green et al. 1970; Mason et al. 1997; Travis 1994). Such findings support the traditional claim that conscious learning and self-induced plasticity can occur even in the most primary pathways and complexes of the central nervous system (*susumna-nadi-chakra*). They also suggest that normally unconscious behavioral responses can be deconditioned by euphoria-mediated lucid insight.

A likely mechanism for process practices is that prosody- and imagery-mediated activation deepens the lateral hypothalamic driving of septal-hippocampal theta by recruiting pontine neurons that promote REM. This induces a lucid, REM-like state in which prosocial-consummatory emotional response patterns not prefigured in instinctual programs can be rehearsed and consolidated (Gackenbach 1992; Jevning et al. 1992; Loizzo 1998; Panksepp 1998). Within this state, sexual imagery–mediated selective kindling of the ventromedial-hypothalamic consummation system deepens septal euphoria, inducing a lucid orgasm-like euphoric state that supports the deconditioning of addictive-defensive behavioral responses and the learning of consummatory-nurturant alternatives (Doidge 1990; Halper 1998; Krivan et al.

1995; Loizzo 1998; Mandell 1979; Mason et al. 1997). In sum, high-arousal heightening of attention in primary process practices appears to result from manipulations that deepen limbic-hypothalamic reward activation. These manipulations also recruit the extrapyramidal–basal ganglia axis (the reptilian brain) for behaviorally enriched learning (rehearsal and commitment) by activating ventral hypothalamic inhibition of addictive (dopaminergic) seeking and compulsive (noradrenergic) defensiveness that maintain behavioral allostatic load (Bushell 1998; Harte et al. 1995; O'Halloran et al. 1985; Panksepp 1998).

Research, Teaching, and Clinical Uses of Meditation

Beyond its relevance to the biology of self-regulation, meditation plays a key role in neuroscience because it is the best available method of training reliable expert subjects for studies of mind-brain interactions (Austin 1998; Goleman 1977; Ornstein 1972). Varela et al. (1996) argue that cognitive neuroscience lacks a methodology to research the constructive role of intentional acts in brain development and suggest an enactive neuroscience integrating Indian meditative methods. Walsh (1988) advises that modern science use meditative traditions to develop consciousness disciplines for psychiatry. Others have argued that meditative methods enhance impartial objectivity and empathy gained by a training analysis and thus should be integrated into psychotherapy training (Burnard 1987; Chung 1990; Dubin 1994; Epstein 1995; Santorelli 1999). Still others advocate using mindfulness in the medical curriculum (Santorelli 1999; S. Shapiro et al. 1998; Sommer and Hassed 1995) and in science in general (Delmonte 1987; Wicklund 1975).

As for clinical indications, some have concluded that, in mind-body therapies, the conventional disease-based treatment approach should be complemented by a skills-learning positive health approach (Ryff and Singer 1998). This conclusion fits with current research showing the general health benefits of meditation (Goleman and Gurin 1993; Kabat-Zinn 1990) and also fits with the growing number of healthy Americans who meditate. Awareness of the potential health benefits of yoga and meditation has grown with the generation exposed in their youth to Indian traditions (Epstein 1995; Goleman 1977; Hassed 1996; Ornish 1998) and with the popular demand for alternative health practices (Eisenberg et al. 1993). The demand for authentic instruction in Asian meditations has obviated the need for clinical forms of TM (Benson et al. 1975; Carrington 1978), yet the conventional view of the predisposing variables and clinical benefits of meditation still assumes the TM-based view of meditation as a unitary relaxation technique (Carrington 1987; Delmonte 1989; West 1987). This TM-based view sees predisposition to meditative practice in terms of suggestibility and limits its benefits to self-regulation of arousal variables that fuel stress-related physical and mental problems (Craven 1989; Snaith 1998). This TM-based view has given way to typologies of meditation informed by Indian traditions and organized around a new view of meditation as an attentional discipline (Goleman 1977; Kutz et al. 1985). The new view explains the diversity of traditional practices and expands the range of individuals and problems for which meditation may be indicated (Bogart 1991; Kelly 1996). This new view found support in studies showing that traditional mindfulness meditation is well tolerated by the general population and generally effective in conditions in which attention may be a critical variable in cognitive-behavioral change (Kabat-Zinn et al. 1985, 1987, 1992; Teasdale et al. 1995). This new view also predicts responses to different techniques by measuring the predisposition to mental versus somatic anxiety (Davidson et al. 1976) and helps explain the efficacy of traditional practices with techniques for diverse dispositions (Kabat-Zinn et al. 1997).

The framework of meditation I explore in this chapter extends this new view of meditation as attentional discipline and attempts to schematize the spectrum of Indian mind-body health traditions. Because these traditions include elaborate systems of positive health, they appeal to many individuals who use psychotherapy for self-exploration and self-change (Epstein 1990; Kelly 1996; Snaith 1998; Walsh 1988). Similar to our psychotherapy tradition (only older and more cross-cultural), Indo-Asian meditation traditions include a broad array of practices to suit the needs of di-

Table 4–3. Comparative typology of meditative therapies and psychotherapies

Hindu	Buddhist	Analytic	Behavioral
Individual practices	**Low arousal**	**Exclusive attention**	**Cognitive learning**
Hatha yoga	Basic mindfulness	Psychodynamic	Relaxation techniques
TM 1 and 4	Basic shamatha	Ego psychology	Autogenic training
Krishnamurti	Basic vipassana	Classical analysis	Cognitive-behavioral therapy
Social practices	**Low arousal**	**Inclusive attention**	**Affective learning**
Yoga 1 and 2	Giving and taking	Object-relations	Family therapy
Bhakti-Seva	Mind reform	Interpersonal	Dialectical behavior therapy
Vedanta	Zazen/Vipasyana	Existential	Bereavement work
Process practices	**High arousal**	**Integrative attention**	**Behavioral learning**
Yoga 5	Kriya/Carya Tantra	Kohutian	Hypnotherapy
TM 3/yoga 6	Yoga/Anuttarayoga 1	Jungian	Guided imagery
Kundalini/yoga 7	Anuttara yoga tantra 2a	Reichian	Sex therapy
Sahaja/yoga 8	Anuttara yoga tantra 2b/	Lacanian	Intimacy work
	Mahamudra		

Note. TM = transcendental meditation.

verse populations. Meditation traditions also systematized their techniques for professional use in university-based medical and psychologic disciplines (Loizzo and Blackhall 1998; Thurman 1984; V. Wallace 1996; Zysk 1991). By comparing these systems with current neuroscience, it should be possible to match dispositions and problems with specific techniques. The framework discussed above suggests a preliminary typology (Table 4–3). This typology assumes a structural-developmental perspective and maps techniques in terms of learning-related variables in cognitive, affective, and behavioral dimensions. In what follows, I offer some general guidelines for the clinical uses of meditation following the typology derived from the learning-based framework of meditation discussed earlier in this chapter.

Meditation may be of interest and benefit to anyone wishing to take an active role in his or her psychiatric care or psychotherapy or in promoting mental health (Delmonte 1984d, 1987, 1988; Kelly 1996; Kutz et al. 1985; W. Smith et al. 1995). Similar to free association, meditative introspection routinely heightens awareness of anxiety, negative emotions, traumatic memories, and derealizing experiences, such as hypnagogic illusions, and thus may make patients more aware of their symptoms (Lazarus 1976; Walsh and Roche 1979; West 1987). In meditation traditions, as in psychotherapy, care is taken to prepare individuals, especially early meditators, with cognitive strategies that foster insight and self-control (Barbieri 1996; Castillo 1990; A. Wallace 1999). Selecting a practice appropriate to individual objectives, level of development, character style, and/or psychopathology is also crucial to long-term success (Engler 1984; D. Shapiro 1992). Given an open mindset and setting, meditation is well tolerated even by individuals with major psychiatric disorders, the largest problem usually being compliance (Delmonte 1984b, 1988; Luckoff et al. 1986). Although meditation has been beneficial in recovery from chemical dependency (Benson and Wallace 1971; Brautigam 1977; Murphy et al. 1986; Schafii et al. 1974, 1975; Shaffer et al. 1997), most instructors advise those actively abusing substances that 1–6 months of sobriety is a prerequisite for stable practice (Kabat-Zinn 1982). Traditionally, people with acute illnesses or exposed to extreme environmental stressors are advised to stabilize their condition and minimize exposure before learning to meditate (MacDonald 1977). Yet these contraindications are relative, and the current consensus is that predisposition and motivation, rather than the nature or severity of symptoms or circumstances, most determine the ability to sustain an effective meditation practice (Delmonte 1981, 1984d, 1995; Kabat-Zinn et al. 1985). Some argue that meditation works best for milder symptoms (Delmonte 1984b, 1988), but this argument overlooks the effectiveness of traditional multicomponent approaches and neglects advanced techniques (Kabat-Zinn 1990; Linehan 1993). Refractory illnesses and severe stress often provide the incentive to meditate, a basic fact of life to which the traditional systems are well adapted (Epstein 1995; Kabat-Zinn 1990; Mikulas 1978; West 1987).

As for specific techniques, individual self-healing practices, such as basic mindfulness, vipassana, basic TM, hatha yoga, basic quiescence meditation, tai chi, martial arts, and clinical meditations, are best suited to high-anxiety, high-control individuals with low stress tolerance, low affect tolerance, at least moderate self-esteem, and moderate capacity for attentional absorption (Delmonte 1984a, 1987, 1988, 1995; Dinardo and Raymond 1979; Hjelle 1974; Spanos et al. 1980; Turnbull and Norris 1982). Individual practices have been found effective for adjustment to general stressors (Beauchamp-Turner and Levinson 1992; Easterlin and Cardena 1998), anxiety and obsessional conditions (Benson and Wallace 1971; Castillo 1990; Girodo 1974; Kabat-Zinn et al. 1992), acute traumatic stress (Miller 1993; Shannahoff-Khalsa and Beckett 1996), and obsessive, avoidant, and sociopathic personality styles (Bleick and Abrams 1987; Fehr 1977; Orme-Johnson et al. 1977; J. Smith 1978). They have also been found effective for somatization, chronic pain, and chemical dependency (Kabat-Zinn et al. 1985; Murthy et al. 1997; Shaffer et al. 1997). As adjunctive therapies, individual practices may work best with dynamic therapies (Bogart 1991; Delmonte 1995; Epstein 1995; Kutz et al. 1985), CBT (Berwick and Oziel 1973; Mikulas 1981; Teasdale et al. 1995), desensitization (Castillo 1990; Greenwood and Benson 1977), behavioral medicine (Benson et al. 1978; Daniels 1975; Kabat-Zinn et al. 1985), consultation-liaison psychiatry (Glueck and Stroebel 1975; Kabat-Zinn 1982, 1990), and substance abuse counseling (Shaffer et al. 1997; Taub et al. 1994). The best-studied clinical application of these practices has been the use of mindfulness for anxiety disorder. Early studies showed clinical meditation techniques to be as effective as hypnosis and more effective than relaxation for the treatment of anxiety (Benson et al. 1978; Daniels 1975). A study by Kabat-Zinn and colleagues (1992) corrected some of the methodologic problems limiting prior work, including self-selection bias and lack of correction for inconsistencies in self-report versus behavioral measures. This study showed that an 8-week program in mindfulness-based stress reduction has efficacy for anxiety and related depression that is comparable with conventional treatments. A follow-up study demonstrated 4-year stability of effects and distinguished the cognitive-behavioral learning strategy in mindfulness from those in CBT, desensitization, and hypnosis (Miller et al. 1995). Despite the limits of small sample size and lack of randomly selected comparison and control groups, the mindfulness studies further support the growing consensus that individual meditation practices are as effective in treating anxiety as conventional therapies and more effective than relaxation alone.

Social self-transcendence practices, such as self-analytic insight, loving-kindness, Hindu yoga (steps 1 and 2), Hindu devotional practices), Tibetan practices such as giving and taking or mind-training, and East Asian Buddhist practices such as Zazen, are suited to interpersonally sensitive individuals with social anxiety, low role-stress tolerance, and moderate affect tolerance and absorption capacity (Heide et al. 1980; Lesh 1970; Maupin 1965; J. Smith 1987; Tloczynski and Tantriella 1998). Studies have suggested that these practices are effective for adjustment to social stressors (Sasaki 1992; Tloczynski and Tantriella 1998); social anxiety (Fergusson and Gowan 1976; Maupin 1965); depressive disorders (Edwards 1997); the sequelae of physical and sexual abuse (Linehan 1993; Linehan and Shearin 1988); depressive, paranoid, and borderline personality styles (Linehan et al. 1992; Simpson et al. 1998; Sweet 1990); and relationship dependency (Linehan 1993; Sweet 1990). As adjuncts, social self-transcendence practices may work best in conjunction with object-relational (Finn 1992; Leone 1995), interpersonal (Newman 1994), and existential therapies (Aitken 1982; Edwards 1997; Lesh 1970; Welwood 1982); long-term treatment of physical or sexual abuse (Linehan 1993; Simpson et al. 1998); cognitive-behavioral skills groups (Linehan et al. 1979; Simpson et al. 1998; Sweet 1990); and family-marital therapies (Jain et al. 1985). The best-studied use of these practices is in the cognitive-behavioral treatment of borderline personality disorder. Linehan et al. (1979) distinguish the group skills training in dialectical behavior therapy (DBT) from conventional CBT with reference to Zen concepts of interdependence and Zazen meditation. Studies have shown DBT to be superior to conventional psychotherapy in reducing depression, self-injury, and rehospitalization in borderline personality disorder (Linehan and Shearin 1988; Linehan et al. 1991, 1992; Simpson et al. 1998).

Advanced process practices, including Hindu yoga (stages 5–8), kundalini yoga, siddha yoga, sahaja yoga, ananda marga tantric yoga, raja yoga (TM stage 3/TM-Sidhi), Kashmiri Shaivite tantra, Indo-Tibetan Buddhist anuttara yoga tantra, *mahamudra*, or *dzog chen*, may be best suited to high-intensity, low-control individuals with performance anxiety, high stress tolerance, high affect tolerance, and high capacities for expressed emotion, absorption, imagery-mediated mentation and sexual response (Choudhary 1985; Corby et al. 1978; Delmonte 1987; Fehr 1977; Gelderloos et al. 1990; Spanos et al. 1980). Preliminary studies suggest that these practices may be effective for dysthymia (W. Smith et al. 1995; Telles and Naveen 1997); performance anxiety (Fergusson and Gowan 1976); inhibited creativity (Fergusson 1993; Jedrczak et al. 1985); the sequelae of childhood neglect (Abramovitch 1995); bipolar disorder (Gackenbach 1992; Gellhorn and Kiely 1972); histrionic, narcissistic, and schizoid personality styles (Alexander et al. 1991; Gelderloos et al. 1990); and shame-based inhibitions to healthy sexuality and intimacy (Jedrczak et al. 1985; Shapiro and Walsh 1982). As adjuncts, process practices may work best with Kohutian, Jungian, and Reichian analysis (Gottschalk 1989; Jung 1978; Karawatt 1991; Kelly 1996; Spiegelman and Miyuki 1985), guided imagery (Karawatt 1991), psychodrama therapies, hypnotherapies (Marriott 1996), and sexual therapies (Gellhorn and Kiely 1972; Mandell 1979). Work adapting process vehicle techniques to clinical settings and problems has just begun (Katzenstein 1998). Given findings that mental imagery is effective for mood regulation (Kosslyn 1994) and that process techniques reduce seizure activity (Deepak et al. 1994; Panjawani et al. 1996), one promising area for study is the use of process visualization practices in bipolar disorder.

There is a growing body of literature on how meditation affects alliance (Carrington 1984; Epstein 1995; Kennet et al. 1975; Kutz et al. 1985; Moleno 1998; Vigne 1991; Welwood 1982). Because many who use alternative methods assume physicians will be skeptical (Eisenberg et al. 1993; Winterholler et al. 1997), it is incumbent on clinicians to ask patients about alternative methods. We should learn enough to advise patients about the risks and benefits of alternative therapies and whether they complement conventional care. Growing consensus on the safety and general health benefits of meditation makes it reasonable for clinicians to support and monitor its use by most patients. When meditation seems to conflict with treatment, there is a sizable amount of literature in which clinicians familiar with meditative traditions explore areas of agreement and clash with psychotherapy (Bogart 1991; Claxton 1986; Epstein 1988, 1990, 1995; Gregoire 1990; Moleno 1998). The difference in approaches to alliance in meditative and psychotherapy traditions is more problematic (Cooper 1999; Kennet et al. 1975; Welwood 1982). Meditation ultimately involves self-reliance, but in practice, critical reliance on a teacher, expert guide, or mentor is considered the most effective means of progress, especially for the advanced meditator (Thurman 1984, 1998). The relationships in meditation practice are more tutorial in nature, resembling the empathic encounter favored by Jung, Ferenczi, Winnicott, and Kohut. Another distinctive feature of meditative alliance is the importance placed on the real relationship, especially on the student's responsibility for choosing a teacher who can model desired qualities. Although these features appear to burden the clinician, the relationship in meditative therapies is often more collegial than in conventional therapies, perhaps because vulnerability and responsibility are more shared (Santorelli 1999; Welwood 1982). The positive health bias of meditative therapies may heighten therapeutic optimism and challenge the alliance, but meditative traditions recognize the depth of resistance and base their optimism on depth-analytic methods and empathic skills that may help correct the pathologizing bias of disease-based conventional care (Cooper 1999; S. Shapiro et al. 1998).

The course and outcome of meditative therapies can vary widely depending on the individual, the objectives, and the practice involved (Engler 1984; D. Shapiro 1992; Walsh 1988). In contrast to clinical meditations, traditional meditations are viewed less as isolated techniques than as the deepest forms of life learning (Thurman 1984). This insight-oriented, long-term process approach resembles that in analytic therapies (Epstein 1995; Moleno 1998). Like psychotherapy, meditation can be practiced with very modest objectives, as in Indo-Tibetan medical traditions in which it is part of multicomponent lifestyle therapies (Loizzo and Blackhall 1998; Ornish et al. 1990). Even a short course of lifestyle therapy can have profound, lasting effects and better outcomes than conventional treatments (Kabat-Zinn 1982; Kabat-Zinn et al. 1985, 1987). Selective use of meditation techniques to complement conventional treatments is feasible provided that the multicomponent lifestyle approach is respected (Linehan 1993). Outcome studies suggest that meditation may have long-term trait-changing effects, not just as the result of repeated state change but also by the incorporation of meditative insights and skills into nonmeditative activities in daily life (Davidson and Goleman 1977; Kabat-Zinn et al. 1987). More than mere attentional alterations, meditative lifestyle therapies involve alterations in cognitive and affective problem solving combined with alternative behavioral strategies that foster an internally enriched learning environment (Loizzo 1998; Rubin 1985; Warrenburg and Pagano 1983).

Over the years, evidence has been mounting that meditation-based mind-body methods enhance health care satisfaction and have the potential to cut medical costs (Benson 1996). The consensus is reflected in the recent NIH initiative to fund mind-body medical centers. Of the many factors contributing to the effect of meditative therapies on health care, three are especially relevant to psychiatry. One factor is patient satisfaction with meditative therapies, thought to be related to increased self-control (Austin 1997; Dinardo and Raymond 1979; Kabat-Zinn et al. 1987; Pelletier 1997; Stek and Bass 1973). This results from the learning of concepts and skills that support a more active role in self-care and treatment (Snaith 1998). A second factor is a product of this enhanced self-regulation (Barbieri 1996). Studies showing that patients with chronic pain, anxiety, personality, and psychotic disorders need less psychotropic medications when they meditate suggest that meditative methods may be useful complements to psychopharmacology, especially in cases of resistance, toxicity or patient preference (Kabat-Zinn 1982; Kabat-Zinn et al. 1985; Miller et al. 1995; Shanahoff-Khalsa and Beckett 1996). Finally, meditative therapies can help fill the gap between clinical needs and fiscal constraints, because they supplement individual therapies with educational groups and self-care practices in an intensive lifestyle modality that helps clinicians do more with less, even in the face of the difficult problems posed by patients with chronic pain and BPD (Kabat-Zinn et al. 1987; Linehan 1993; Simpson et al. 1998; Urbanowski and Miller 1996).

How do meditative therapies compare with conventional psychotherapies? In the Indo-Tibetan synthesis, all three vehicles of meditative practice are viewed as part of a single developmental continuum of practice, whose three vehicles are likened to a family born of one mother (self-analytic insight) and three fathers (renunciative, empathic, and impassioned techniques) (Thurman 1998). This synthesis helps explain why Asian meditative practices have been compared with so many different therapies (Benson et al. 1978; Epstein 1995; Kabat-Zinn 1982; Linehan 1993; Snaith 1998). Here, I can only touch on basic resemblances and direct the reader to references for distinctions. Like cognitive therapies and desensitization, this tradition sees behavior as more or less ingrained habitual action, reinforced by conditioning and modifiable by learning (Kabat-Zinn et al. 1985; Mikulas 1981; Teasdale et al. 1995). Like classical analytic and dynamic therapies, it sees the learning process as limited by cognitive and affective resistances to insight, that is, self-deceptive defenses shaped by development and rooted in evolutionary egocentric instincts (Emavardhana and Tori 1997; Epstein 1988; Moleno 1998). Like object-relations and interpersonal therapies, it sees human nature as fundamentally social and locates development within a naturally constructive social field (Engler 1984; Finn 1992; Hayward 1998; Linehan 1993). Like focusing and autogenic therapy, it uses attentional alterations to enhance problem-solving and emotional self-regulation (Snaith 1998). Like Jungian analysis and hypnotherapy, it uses imagery-mediated insight and attentional absorption to expose and reform self-object constructs (Karawatt 1991; Spiegelman and Miyuki 1994). Like Reichian analysis and sexual therapies, it uses sexual arousal and euphoria-mediated insight to disarm behavioral defenses and enhance mind-body openness (Kahn 1985). Although Asian meditative traditions will never be all things to all people, as some seem to suggest, one of their lasting contributions may be their mature integration of divergent therapeutic paradigms that are only gradually being reconciled in contemporary psychiatry.

Of course, the framework and guidelines developed in this chapter must be regarded as provisional, based as they are on preliminary data and findings from related fields. Yet the consensus on meditation is clearer and more evidence-based than on most complementary therapies, and the need for coherent clinical guidelines is pressing enough that some interpretative framework is warranted, however speculative and provisional. The long-term prescription is further research. Given the recent NIH initiative on mind-body medicine, the prospects are good for a more definitive framework and guidelines on meditative therapies. The comparative approach of this chapter accords with D. Shapiro's (1987) recommendation that meditation research be treated as a subset of psychotherapy research. However, it adds to his methodological reasons the mechanistic considerations and comparative learning model of meditation discussed above. This addition is not insignificant, because the model coordinates traditional learning models of meditation with new approaches to psychopathology and psychotherapy based on the neuroscience of stress, learning, and neural plasticity and on related concepts of allostasis and environmental enrichment. The model establishes linkages between the three phases of the stress response, three degrees of allostatic load, three levels of stress-induced psychopathology, three structural-functional mechanisms of enriched learning, three vehicles of meditative practice, and three main types of therapies. It is hoped that this model will stimulate research, serve as an educational aid, and offer provisional guidelines for clinicians facing a challenging yet exciting new field in psychiatry.

References

Abramovitch H: The nightmare of returning home: a case of acute onset nightmare disorder treated by lucid dreaming. Isr J Psychiatry Relat Sci 32:140–145, 1995

Adey W, Bell F, Dennis B: Effects of LSD, psilocibin and psilocin on temporal lobe EEG patterns in the cat. Neurology 12:591–602, 1962

Aitken R: Zen practice and psychotherapy. Journal of Transpersonal Psychology 14:18–22, 1982

Alexander C, Rainforth M, Maxwell V, et al: Transcendental meditaton, self-actualization, and psychological health: a conceptual overview and meta-analysis. Journal of Social Behavior and Personality 6:189–248, 1991

Anand B, Chinna G, Singh B: Some aspects of electroencephalographic studies in yogis. Electroencephalogr Clin Neurophysiol 13:452–456, 1961

Austin J: Stress reduction through mindfulness meditation: effects on psychological symptomatology, sense of control, and spiritual experiences. Psychother Psychosom 66:97–106, 1997

Austin J: Zen and the Brain: Toward an Understanding of Meditation and Consciousness. Cambridge, MA, MIT Press, 1998

Bagchi B, Wegner M: Electrophysiological correlates of some yogi exercises. Electroencephalogr Clin Neurophysiol Suppl 7:132–149, 1957

Banquet J: EEG in meditation. Electroencephalogr Clin Neurophysiol 35:143–151, 1973

Barbieri P: Confronting stress: integrating control theory and mindfulness to cultivate our inner resources through mind-body methods. Journal of Reality Therapy 15:3–13, 1996

Barr D, Lambert N, Hoyt K, et al: Induction and reversal of long term potentiation by low and high intensity theta pattern stimulation. J Neurosci 15:5402–5410, 1995

Baumgartner J, Epstein C: Voluntary alteration of visual evoked potentials. Ann Neurol 12:475–478, 1982

Bear D, Freeman R, Schiff D, et al: Interictal behavioral changes in patients with temporal lobe epilepsy, in Annual Review of Neuropsychiatry. Washington DC, American Psychiatric Association, 1985, pp 190–214

Beary J, Benson H: A simple psychophysiologic technique which elicits the hypometabolic changes of the relaxation response. Psychosom Med 36:115–120, 1974

Beauchamp-Turner D, Levinson D: Effects of meditation on stress, health, and affect. Med Psychother Internat J 5:123–131, 1992

Beck A, Rush A, Shaw B, et al: Cognitive Therapy of Depression. New York, Guilford, 1979

Benson H: Systematic hypertension and the relaxation response. N Engl J Med 296:1152–1156, 1977

Benson H: Mind over maladies: can yoga, prayer, and meditation be adapted for managed care? Hosp Health Netw 70:26–27, 1996

Benson H, Wallace R: Decreased drug abuse with transcendental meditation: a study of 1,862 subjects, in Congressional Record, 92nd Congress, 1st Session, Serial No. 92-1. Washington, DC, U.S. Government Printing Office, 1971

Benson H, Wallace R: Decreased blood pressure in hypertensive subjects who practice meditation. Circulation 45(suppl 2):516, 1972

Benson H, Alexander S, Feldman C: Decreased premature ventricular contractions through the use of the relaxation response in patients with stable ischemic heart disease. Lancet 2:380–382, 1975

Benson H, Frankel F, Apfel R, et al: Treatment of anxiety: a comparison of the usefulness of self-hypnosis and a meditational relaxation technique. Psychother Psychosom 30:229–242, 1978

Benson H, Lehman J, Malhotra M, et al: Body temperature changes during the practice of gTummo heat yoga. Nature 295:234–236, 1982

Benson H, Malhotra M, Goldman R, et al: Three case reports of the metabolic and electroencephalographic changes during advanced Buddhist meditative techniques. Behav Med 16:90–95, 1990

Berkenwald AD: In the name of medicine. Ann Intern Med 128:246–250, 1998

Berwick P, Oziel L: The use of meditation as a behavioral technique. Behav Ther 4:743–745, 1973

Bleick C, Abrams A: The transcendental meditation program and criminal recidivism in California. Journal of Criminal Justice 15:211–230, 1987

Block B: The use of transcendental meditation as a reciprocal inhibitor in psychotherapy. J Psychother 9:78–82, 1977

Bogart G: The use of meditation in psychotherapy: a review of the literature. Am J Psychother 45:382–412, 1991

Bradwejn J, Dowdall M, Iny L, et al: Can East and West meet in psychoanalysis? Am J Psychiatry 142:1226–1228, 1985

Brautigam E: Effects of the transcendental meditation program on drug abusers: a prospective study, in Scientific Research on the Transcendental Meditation Program. Edited by Orme-Johnson D, Farrow J. Los Angeles, CA, Maharishi University Press, 1977, pp 506–514

Bremner J, Randall P, Scott T, et al: MRI-based measurement of hippocampal volume in patients with combat-related post-traumatic stress disorder. Am J Psychiatry 1527:973–981, 1995

Brown D: A model for the levels of concentrative meditation. Int J Clin Exp Hypn 25:236–273, 1977

Brown D, Forte M, Dysart M: Differences in visual sensitivity among mindfulness meditators and non-meditators. Percept Mot Skills 58:727–733, 1984

Burnard P: Meditation: uses and methods in psychiatric nurse education. Nurs Educ Today 7:187–191, 1987

Bushell W: Imagery, bliss and healing in the Indo-Tibetan unexcelled yoga tantras. Paper presented at the First International Congress on Tibetan Medicine. Washington DC, Georgetown Medical School, October, 1998

Carney N, Chestnut R, Maynard H, et al: Effect of cognitive rehabilitation on outcomes of persons with traumatic brain injury. J Head Trauma Rehabil 14:277–303, 1999

Carrington P: Clinically Standardized Meditation (CSM) Instructor's Kit. Kendall Park, NJ, Pace Educational Systems, 1978

Carrington P: Releasing. New York, William Morrow, 1984

Carrington P: Managing meditation in clinical practice, in The Psychology of Meditation. Edited by West M. Oxford, England, Clarendon Press, 1987, pp 150–172

Carroll B: Psychopathology and neurobiology of manic-depressive disorders, in Psychopathology and the Brain. Edited by Carroll B, Barrett J. New York, Raven, 1991, pp 265–285

Castillo R: Depersonalization and meditation. Psychiatry 53:158–168, 1990

Choudhary K: Meditation and tantra: a psychiatric perspective. Dynamische Psychiatrie 18:276–282, 1985

Chung C: Psychotherapist and expansion of awareness. Psychother Psychosom 53:28–32, 1990

Ciringotta F, Todesco C, Lugaresi E: Case report: temporal lobe epilepsy with ecstatic seizures (so called Dosteyevsky epilepsy). Epilepsia 21:705–710, 1980

Claxton G (ed): Beyond Psychotherapy: The Impact of Eastern Religions on Psychological Theory and Practice. London, England, Wisdom Publications, 1986

Claxton G: Meditation in Buddhist psychology, in The Psychology of Meditation. Edited by West M. Oxford, England, Clarendon Press, 1987, pp 23–38

Cooper P: Buddhist meditation and countertransference: a case study. Am J Psychoanal 59:71–85, 1999

Coplan J, Andrews MW, Gorman J, et al: Persistent elevations of CSF concentration of corticotropin releasing hormone in adult non-human primates exposed to early life stressors. Proc Natl Acad Sci U S A 93:1619–1623, 1996

Corby J, Roth W, Zarcone V, et al: Psychophysiological correlates of the practice of tantric yoga meditation. Arch Gen Psychiatry 35:571–577, 1978

Craven J: Meditation and psychotherapy. Can J Psychiatry 34:648–653, 1989

Crawford H, Meszaros I, Szabo C: EEG differences in low and high hypnotizables during waking and hypnosis: rest, math and imaginal tasks, in Hypnosis. Edited by Peterson D, Wilkie E. London, England, Whurr Publishers, 1989, pp 31–40

Daniels L: The treatment of psychophysiological disorders and severe anxiety by behavior therapy, hypnosis, and transcendental meditation. Am J Clin Hypnos 17:267–269, 1975

Darnell A, Bremner J, Licino J, et al: CSF levels of corticortopin releasing factor in chronic posttraumatic stress disorder. Neuroscience Abstracts 20:15, 1994

Das N, Gastaut H: Variations de l'activite electrique de cerveau du coeur et des muscles squelletiques au cours de la meditation et de l'extase yogique. Electroencephalogr Clin Neurophysiol Suppl 6:211–219, 1955

Davidson R: The physiology of meditation and mystical states of consciousness. Perspect Biol Med 19:345–380, 1976

Davidson R, Goleman D: The role of attention in meditation and hypnosis: a psychobiological perspective on transformations of consciousness. Int J Clin Exp Hypn 25:291–308, 1977

Davidson R, Goleman D, Schwartz G: Attentional and affective concomitants of meditation. J Abnorm Psychol 85:235–238, 1976

Deepak K, Manchanda S, Maheshwari M: Meditation improves clinicoencephalographic measures in drug-resistant epileptics. Biofeedback and Self-Regulation 19:25–40, 1994

Deikman A: Deautomatisation and the mystic experience. Psychiatry 29:481–489, 1966

Delmonte M: Suggestibility and meditation. Psychol Rep 48:727–737, 1981

Delmonte M: Factors influencing the regularity of meditation practice in a clinical population. Br J Med Psychol 57:275–278, 1984a

Delmonte M: Meditation: some similarities with hypnoidal states and hypnosis. International Journal of Psychosomatics 31:24–34, 1984b

Delmonte M: Physiological concomitants of meditation practice: a literature review. International Journal of Psychosomatics 31:35–36, 1984c

Delmonte M: Psychometric scores and meditation practice: a literature review. Personal and Individual Differences 5:559–563, 1984d

Delmonte M: Biochemical indices associated with meditation practice: a literature review. Neurosci Biobehav Rev 9:557–561, 1985

Delmonte M: Personality and meditation, in The Psychology of Meditation. Edited by West M. Oxford, England, Clarendon, 1987, pp 118–131

Delmonte M: Personality correlates of meditation practice and frequency in an outpatient population. J Behav Med 11:593–597, 1988

Delmonte M: Meditation, the unconscious, and psychosomatic disorders. International Journal of Psychosomatics 36:45–52, 1989

Delmonte M: Meditation and the unconscious. Journal of Contemporary Psychotherapy 25:223–242, 1995

DePascalis V, Penna P: 40-Hz EEG acitivity during hypnotic induction and hypnotic testing. Int J Clin Exp Hypn 38:125–138, 1990

Dinardo P, Raymond J: Locus of control and attention during meditation. J Consult Clin Psychol 47:1136–1137, 1979

Drevets WC, Videen TO, Price JL, et al: A functional anatomical study of unipolar depression. J Neurosci 12:3628–3641, 1992

Doidge N: Appetitive pleasure states: a biopsychoanalytic model of the pleasure threshold, mental representation and defense, in Pleasure Beyond the Pleasure Principle. Edited by Glick R, Bone S. New Haven, CT, Yale University Press, 1990, pp 138–173

Dubin W: The use of meditative techniques in teaching dynamic psychotherapy. Journal of Transpersonal Psychology 26:19–36, 1994

Earle J: Cerebral laterality and meditation: a review, in Meditation: Classics and Contemporary Perspectives. Edited by Shapiro D, Walsh R. New York, Aldine Publishing, 1984, pp 171–190

Easterlin B, Cardena E: Cognitive and emotional differences between short- and long-term Vipassana meditators. Imagination, Cognition, and Personality 18:69–81, 1998

Edwards M: Being present: experiential connections between Zen Buddhist practices and the grieving process. Disabil Rehabil 19:44–51, 1997

Eisenberg DR, Kessler RC, Foster C, et al: Unconventional medicine in the United States: prevalence, costs and patterns of use. N Engl J Med 328:246–252, 1993.

Emavardhana T, Tori C: Changes in self-concept, ego defense mechanisms, and religiosity following seven-day Vipassana meditation retreats. Journal of the Scientific Study of Religion 36:194–206, 1997

Engler J: Therapeutic aims in psychotherapy and meditation: developmental stages in the representation of self. Journal of Transpersonal Psychology 16:80–93, 1984

Epstein M: The deconstruction of the self: ego and "egolessness" in Buddhist insight meditation. Journal of Transpersonal Psychology 20:61–69, 1988

Epstein M: Beyond the oceanic feeling: psychoanalytic study of Buddhist meditation. International Review of Psychoanalysis 17:159–166, 1990

Epstein M: Thoughts Without a Thinker. San Francisco, CA, Harper Collins, 1995

Erlichman H, Weiner M: EEG asymmetry during covert mental activity. Psychophysiology 17:228–235, 1980

Farmer J, Clippard D: Educational outcomes in children with disabilities. Neurorehabilitation 5:49–56, 1994

Farrow J, Herbert J: Breath suspension during the transcendental meditation technique. Psychosom Med 44:133–153, 1982

Fawcett J: Suicide risk factors in depressive disorders and panic disorder. J Clin Psychiatry 53:9–13, 1992

Fehr T: A longitudinal study of the effect of transcendental meditation program on changes in personality, in Scientific Research on the Transcendental Meditation Program. Edited by Orme-Johnson D, Farrow J. Los Angeles, CA, Maharishi University Press, 1977, pp 476–483

Fenwick P: Meditation and the EEG, in The Psychology of Meditation. Edited by West M. Oxford, England, Clarendon Press, 1987, pp 104–117

Ferchmin P, Ertovic V: Forty minutes of experience increase the weight and RNA content of cerebral cortex in preadolescent rats. Dev Psychobiol 19:511–519, 1989

Fergusson L: Field independence, transcendental meditation, and achievement in college art: a reexamination. Percept Mot Skills 77:1104–1106, 1993

Fergusson L, Gowan J: TM: Some preliminary psychological findings. Journal of Humanistic Psychology 16:51–60, 1976

Fieve R: Bipolar II disorder and its proposed beneficial subtype bipolar IIb: a desirable disorder? in Current Psychiatric Therapy II. Edited by Dunner D. Philadelphia, PA, WB Saunders, 1997, pp 261–266

Finn M: Transitional space and Tibetan Buddhism: the object relations of meditation, in Object Relations Theory and Religion. Edited by Finn M, Gartner J. Westport, Praeger, 1992, pp 109–118

Fugh-Berman A: Alternative Medicine: What Works. Tucson, AZ, Odonian Press, 1996

Funderburk J: Science Studies Yoga: A Review of Physiological Data. Himalayan Institute, 1977

Gackenbach J: Interhemispheric EEG coherence in REM sleep and meditation: the lucid dreaming connection, in The Neuropsychology of Sleep and Dreaming. Edited by Antrobus J, Bertini M. Hillsdale, NJ, Erlbaum, 1992, pp 265–288

Gelderloos P, Hermans F, Ahlscrom H, et al: Transcendence and psychological health: studies with long-term participants of the transcendental meditation and TM-Sidhi program. Journal of Psychology 124:177–197, 1990

Gellhorn E, Kiely W: Mystical states of consciousness: neurophysiological and clinical aspects. J Nerv Ment Dis 154:399–405, 1972

Gimello R: Mysticism and meditation, in Mysticism and Philosophical Analysis. Edited by Katz S. Oxford, England, Oxford University Press, 1978, pp 170–199

Girodo M: Yoga meditation and flooding in the treatment of anxiety neurosis. J Behav Ther Exp Psychiatry 5:157–160, 1974

Glueck B, Stroebel C: Biofeedback and meditation in the treatment of psychiatric illness. Compr Psychiatry 16:303–321, 1975

Goleman D: The Varieties of Meditative Experience. New York, Dutton, 1977

Goleman D, Gurin J: Mind-Body Medicine. New York, Consumer Reports Books, 1993

Gottschalk L: How to Do Self-Analysis and Other Self-Psychotherapies. Northvale, Jason Aronson, 1989

Govinda A: The Psychological Attitude of Early Buddhist Philosophy and Its Systematic Representation According to Abhidhamma Tradition. New York, Samuel Weiser, 1974

Green E, Ferguson A, Green A, et al: Preliminary Report on Voluntary Controls Project: Swami Rama. Topeka, KS, Menninger Foundation, 1970

Greenough W, Volkmar F: Pattern of dendritic branching in occipital cortex of rats reared in complex environments. Exp Neurol 40:136–143, 1973

Greenwood M, Benson H: The efficacy of progressive relaxation in systematic desensitization and a proposal for an alternative competitive response—the relaxation response. Behav Res Ther 15:337–343, 1977

Gregoire J: Therapy with a person who meditates: diagnosis and treatment strategies. Transactional Analysis Journal 20:60–76, 1990

Gruzelier J, Brow T: Psychophysiological evidence for a state theory of hypnosis and susceptibility. J Psychosom Res 29:287–302, 1985

Haddjeri N, Seletti B, Gilbert F, et al: Effect of ergotamine on serotonin-modulated responses in the rodent and human brain. Neuropsychopharmacology 19:365–380, 1998

Halper J: Advanced Buddhist meditation and the internal reward system. Paper presented at the First International Congress on Tibetan Medicine. Washington, DC, Georgetown Medical School, October, 1998

Harte J, Eifert G, Smith R: The effects of running and meditation on beta-endorphin, corticotropin-releasing hormone and cortisol in plasma, and on mood. Biol Psychiatry 40:251–265, 1995

Hassed C: Meditation in general practice. Aust Fam Physician 25:1257–1260, 1996

Hayward J: A dzogs-chen Buddhist interpretation of the sense of self. Journal of Consciousness Studies 5:611–626, 1998

Heath R: Electrical self-stimulation in the brain of man. Am J Psychiatry 120:571–577, 1963

Heide F, Wadlington W, Lundy R: Hypnotic responsivity as a predictor of outcome in meditation. Int J Clin Exp Hypn 28:358–366, 1980

Heller C, Elsner R, Rao N: Voluntary hypometabolism in an Indian Yogi. Journal of Thermal Biology 2:171–173, 1987

Herzog H, Lele V, Kuwert K, et al: Changed pattern of regional glucose metabolism during yoga meditative relaxation. Neuropsychobiology 23:182–187, 1991

Hjelle L: Transcendental meditation and psychological health. Percept Mot Skills 39:623–628, 1974

Holmes D: The influence of meditation versus rest on physiological arousal: a second examination, in The Psychology of Meditation. Edited by West M. Oxford, England, Clarendon Press, 1987, pp 81–103

Hyman S, Nestler E: Initiation and adaptation: a paradigm for understanding psychotropic drug action. Am J Psychiatry 154:440–441, 1997

Ikemi A: Psychophysiological effects of self-regulation method: EEG frequency analysis and contingent negative variations. Psychother Psychosom 49:230–239, 1988

Infante J, Peran F, Martinez M, et al: ACTH and beta-endorphin in transcendental meditation. Physiol Behav 64:311–315, 1998

Isayeva N: From Early Vedanta to Kashmiri Shaivism. Albany, State University of New York Press, 1995

Jain S, Boswell E, Jain S: Hypnosis, biofeedback, and meditation as adjunctive techniques in treating distressed families. Revista Internazionale di Psicologia e Ipnosi 26:337–345, 1985

Jedrczak A, Beresford M, Clements G: The TM-Sidhi program, pure consciousness, creativity and intelligence. Journal of Creativity and Behavior 19:270–275, 1985

Jella S, Shannahoff-Khalsa D: The effects of forced nostril breathing on cognitive performance. Int J Neurosci 73:61–68, 1993

Jevning R, Wallace R, Beidebach M: The physiology of meditation: a review. A wakeful hypometabolic integrated response. Neurosci Biobehav Rev 16:415–424, 1992

Jevning R, Anand R, Biedenbach M, et al: Effects on regional cerebral bloodflow of transcendental meditation. Physiol Behav 59:339–402, 1996

Jung CG: Psychology and the East. Translated by Hull R. Princeton, NJ, Princeton University Press, 1978

Kabat-Zinn J: An outpatient program based in behavioral medicine for chronic pain patients based on the practice of mindfulness meditation: theoretical considerations and preliminary results. Gen Hosp Psychiatry 4:33–47, 1982

Kabat-Zinn J: Full Catastrophe Living. New York, Bantam, 1990

Kabat-Zinn J, Lipworth L, Burney R: The clinical use of mindfulness meditation for the self-regulation of chronic pain. J Behav Med 8:163–190, 1985

Kabat-Zinn J, Whitworth J, Burney R, et al: Four-year follow up of a meditation-based program for the regulation of chronic pain: treatment outcome and compliance. Clin J Pain 2:159–173, 1987

Kabat-Zinn J, Massion A, Kristeller J, et al: Effectiveness of a meditation-based stress-reduction program in the treatment of anxiety disorders. Am J Psychiatry 149:936–943, 1992

Kabat-Zinn J, Chapman A, Salmon P: Relationship of cognitive and somatic components of anxiety to preference for different relaxation techniques. Mind/Body Medicine 2:101–109, 1997

Kabat-Zinn J, Santorelli S, Salmon P: Effect of mindfulness-based stress-reduction training on stress-mediating trait measures in medical patients: long- and short-term observations. Submitted for publication.

Kagan J, Resnick S, Snidman N: Biological basis of childhood shyness. Science 240:167–171, 1988

Kahn K: Vipassana meditation and the psychobiology of Wilhelm Reich. Journal of Humanistic Psychology 25:117–128, 1985

Kandel E: Biology and the future of psychoanalysis: a new intellectual framework for psychiatry revisited. Am J Psychiatry 156:505–524, 1999

Kandel E, Schwartz J: Principles of Neural Science. New York, Elsevier Science, 1991

Karawatt M: Notes for a study on the active imagination and meditation techniques. Giornale Storico di Psicologia Dinamica 15:31–53, 1991

Kasamatsu A, Harai T: An electroencephalographic study on Zen meditation (zazen). Folia Psychiatr Neurol Jpn 20:315–336, 1966

Kasamatsu A, Okuma T, Takenaka S, et al: The EEG of Zen and yoga practitioners. Electroencepalogr Clin Neurophysiol Suppl 9:51–52, 1957

Katzenstein L: Center for Meditation and Healing integrates psychiatric health. Psychiatric Times 15:1–3, 1998

Kelly G: Using meditative techniques in psychotherapy. Journal of Humanistic Psychology 36:49–66, 1996

Kennet J, Radha S, Frager R: How to be a transpersonal teacher without becoming a guru. Journal of Transpersonal Psychology 7:39–54, 1975

Kissen B: Conscious and Unconscious Programs in the Brain. New York, Plenum, 1986

Kosslyn S: Image and Brain: Resolution of the Imagery Debate. Cambridge, MA, MIT, 1994

Krivan M, Szabo G, Sarnyai Z, et al: Oxytocin blocks the development of heroin-fentanyl cross-tolerance in mice. Pharmacol Biochem Behav 52:591–594, 1995

Kunzendorf R, Shiekh A: Physiology of Mental Imagery. New York, Baywood, 1990

Kutz I, Borysenko J, Benson H: Meditation and psychotherapy: a rationale for the integration of dynamic psychotherapy, the relaxation response and mindfulness meditation. Am J Psychiatry 142:1–8, 1985

Lazarus A: Psychiatric problems precipitated by transcendental meditation. Psychol Rep 39:601–602, 1976

Leone G: Zen meditation: a psychoanalytic conceptualization. Journal of Transpersonal Psychology 27:87–94, 1995

Lesh T: Zen meditation and the development of empathy in counselors. Journal of Humanistic Psychology 10:39–74, 1970

Linehan M: Cognitive Behavioral Treatment of Borderline Personality Disorder. New York, Guilford, 1993

Linehan M, Shearin E: Lethal stress: a social-behavioral model of suicidal behavior, in Handbook of Life Stress, Cognition, and Health. Edited by Fisher S, Reason J. New York, Wiley, 1988, pp 65–285

Linehan M, Goldfried M, Goldfried A: Assertion therapy: skill training or cognitive restructuring. Behavior Therapy 10:372–388, 1979

Linehan M, Armstrong H, Suarez A, et al: Cognitive-behavioral treatment of chronically parasuicidal borderline patients. Arch Gen Psychiatry 48:1060–1064, 1991

Linehan M, Tutek D, Heard H: Interpersonal and social treatment outcomes for borderline personality disorder. Presented at the annual meeting of the Association for the Advancement of Behavior Therapy, Boston, MA, 1992

Liu G, Cui R, Li G, et al: Changes in brainstem and cortical auditory potentials during qi-gong meditation. Am J Chin Med 18:95–103, 1990

Loizzo J: The psychobiology of the Indo-Tibetan unexcelled yoga tantras: a learning model. Paper presented at the First International Congress on Tibetan Medicine. Washington, DC, Georgetown Medical School, October 1998

Loizzo J, Blackhall L: Traditional alternatives as complementary sciences: the case of Indo-Tibetan medicine. J Altern Complement Med 4:311–319, 1998

Luborsky L: Principles of Psychoanalytic Psychotherapy: A Manual for Supportive-Expressive Treatment. New York, Basic Books, 1984

Luckoff D, Wallace C, Liberman R, et al: A holistic program for chronic schizophrenic patients. Schizophr Bull 12:274–282, 1986

MacDonald K: How to Meditate. London, England, Wisdom Books, 1977

MacLean P: The limbic system with respect to two basic life principles, in Second Conference on the Central Nervous System and Behavior. New York, Josiah Macy Foundation, 1959, pp 43–59

Mandell A: Psychiatric aspects of sports. Psychiatric Annals 9:154–160, 1979

Marriott J: Meditation and hypnotherapy. Australian Journal of Clinical Hypnotherapy and Hypnosis 17:53–62, 1996

Mason L, Alexander C, Travis F, et al: Electrophysiological correlates of higher states of consciousness during sleep in long-term practitioners of the transcendental meditation program. Sleep 20:102–110, 1997

Maupin E: Individual differences in response to a Zen meditation exercise. J Clin Consult Psychol 29:139–145, 1965

Mikulas W: Four noble truths of Buddhism related to behavior therapy. Psychological Records 28:59–67, 1978

Mikulas W: Buddhism and behavioral modification. Psychological Records 31:331–342, 1981

Miller J: The unveiling of traumatic memories and emotions through mindfulness and concentration meditation: clinical implications and three case reports. Journal of Transpersonal Psychology 25:169–180, 1993

Miller J, Fletcher K, Kabat-Zinn J: Three-year follow-up and clinical implications of a mindfulness-based stress reduction intervention in the treatment of anxiety disorders. Gen Hosp Psychiatry 17:192–200, 1995

Moleno A: The Couch and the Tree: Dialogues Between Psychoanalysis and Buddhism. New York, North Point Press, 1998

Morse D, Cohen L, Furst L, et al: A physiological evaluation of the yoga concept of respiratory control of autonomic system activity. International Journal of Psychosomatics 31:3–19, 1984

Murphy T, Pagano R, Marlatt G: Lifestyle modification with heavy alcohol drinkers: effects of aerobic exercise and meditation. Addict Behav 11:175–186, 1986

Murthy P, Gangadar B, Janakiranaiah N, et al: Normalization of P300 amplitude following treatment in dysthymia. Biol Psychiatry 42:740–743, 1997

Narayan R, Kamat A, Khanolkar M, et al: Quantitative evaluation of muscle relaxation induced by kundalini yoga with the help of EMG integrator. Indian J Physiol Pharmacol 34:279–281, 1990

Naveen K, Nagarathna R, Nagendra H, et al: Yoga breathing through a particular nostril increases spacial memory scores without lateralized effects. Psychological Reports 81:555–561, 1997

Newman J: Affective empathy training with senior citizens using Zazen meditation. Dissertation Abstracts International Section A 55:1193, 1994

Ng K, Gibbs M: Stages in memory formation: a review, in Neural and Behavioral Plasticity: The Use of the Domestic Chick as a Model. Edited by Andrew R. Oxford, England, Oxford University Press, 1991, pp 351–369

O'Halloran J, Jevning R, Wilson A, et al: Hormonal control in a state of decreased activation: potentiation of argenine vasopressin secretion. Physiol Behav 35:591–595, 1985

Orme-Johnson D: Evidence that transcendental meditation does not produce cognitive kindling: a comment. Percept Mot Skills 81:642, 1995

Orme-Johnson D, Kielbauch J, Moore R, et al: Personality and autonomic changes in prisoners practicing the transcendental meditation technique, in Scientific Research on the Transcendental Meditation Program. Edited by Orme-Johnson D, Farrow J. Los Angeles, CA, Maharishi University Press, 1977, pp 556–561

Ornish D: Love and Survival. San Francisco, CA, Harper Collins, 1998

Ornish D, Brown S, Scherwitz L, et al: Can lifestyle changes reverse coronary heart disease? Lancet 336:129–133, 1990

Ornstein R: The Psychology of Consciousness. San Francisco, CA, WH Freeman, 1972

Panjawani U, Selvamurthy W, Singh S, et al: Effect of Sahaja yoga practice on seizure control and EEG changes in patients with epilepsy. Indian J Med Res 103:165–172, 1996

Panksepp J: Affective Neuroscience. New York, Oxford University Press, 1998

Pelletier K: Effects of the transcendental meditation program on perceptual style: increased field independence, in Scientific Research on the Transcendental Meditation Program. Edited by Orme-Johnson D, Farrow J. Los Angeles, CA, Maharishi University Press, 1977, pp 337–345

Persinger M: Striking EEG profiles from single episodes of glossolalia and transcendental meditation. Percept Mot Skills 58:127–133, 1984

Persinger M: Transcendental meditation and general meditation are associated with enhanced complex partial epileptic-like signs: evidence for "cognitive" kindling? Percept Mot Skills 76:80–82, 1993

Prince R: Meditation: some psychological speculations. Psychology Journal of the University of Ottawa 3:202–209, 1978

Reiser M: Mind, Brain and Body: Toward a Convergence of Psychoanalysis and Neurobiology. New York, Basic Books, 1984

Rosensweig M, Bennett E: Psychobiology of plasticity: effects of training and experienceon brain and behavior. Behav Brain Res 78:57–65, 1996

Rubin J: Meditation and psychoanalytic listening. Psychoanal Rev 72:599–613, 1985

Ryff C, Singer B: The contours of positive human health. Psychological Inquiry 9:1–28, 1998

Sabourin M, Cutomb S, Crawford H, et al: EEG correlates of hypnotic susceptibility and hypnotic trance: spectral analysis and coherence. Int J Psychophysiol 10:125–142, 1990

Santorelli S: Heal Thyself: Lessons on Mindfulness in Medicine. New York, Bell Tower, 1999

Sasaki Y: Developments in Zen therapy based on Zen meditation: an overview. Japanese Psychological Review 35:113–131, 1992

Schacter D: EEG theta waves and psychological phenomena: a review and analysis. Biol Psychol 5:47–82, 1977

Schafii M, Lavely R, Jaffe R: Meditation and marijuana. Am J Psychiatry 131:60–63, 1974

Schafii M, Lavely R, Jaffe R: Meditation and prevention of alcohol abuse. Am J Psychiatry 132:942–945, 1975

Schaie K: The course of adult intellectual development. Am Psychol 49:304–313, 1994

Scherwitz L, Graham L, Grandits G, et al: Self-involvement and coronary heart disease incidence in the Multiple Risk Factor Intervention Trial. Psychosom Med 84:187–199, 1986

Schmidt LA, Fox NA, Rubin KH, et al: Behavioral and neuroendocrine responses in shy children. Dev Psychobiol 30:127–140, 1997

Seeman T, McEwen B, Singer B, et al: Increase in unrinary cortisol excretion and memory declines: MacArthur studies of successful aging. J Clin Endocrinol Metab 82:2458–2465, 1997

Shaffer H, LaSalvia T, Stein J: Comparing hatha yoga with dynamic group psychotherapy for enhancing methadone maintenance treatment: a randomized clinical trial. Alternative Therapies 3:57–66, 1997

Shannahoff-Khalsa D, Beckett L: Clinical case report: efficacy of yogic techniques in the treatment of obsessive compulsive disorders. Int J Neurosci 85:1–17, 1996

Shapiro D: Implications of psychotherapy research for the study of meditation, in The Psychology of Meditation. Edited by West M. Oxford, England, Clarendon, 1987, pp 173–192

Shapiro D: A preliminary study of long-term meditators: goals, effects, religious orientation, cognitions. Journal of Transpersonal Psychology 24:23–39, 1992

Shapiro D, Walsh R: Beyond Health and Normality: Explorations in Exceptional Psychological Well-Being. New York, Van Nostrand, 1982

Shapiro S, Schwartz G, Bonner G: Effects of mindfulness-based stress reduction on medical and premedical students. J Behav Med 21:581–599, 1998

Sheline Y, Wang W, Gado M, et al: Hippocampal atrophy in recurrent unipolar depression. Proc Natl Acad Sci U S A 93:3908–3913, 1996

Shimamura A, Berry J, Mangels J, et al: Memory and cognitive abilities in university professors: evidence for successful aging. Psychological Science 6:271–277, 1995

Shulkin J, McEwen B, Gold P: Allostasis, amygdala, and anticipatory angst. Neurosci Biobehav Rev 18:385–396, 1994

Shulkin J, Gold P, McEwen B: Induction of corticotropin-releasing hormone gene expression by glucocorticoids: implications for understanding the states of fear and anxiety and allostatic load. Psychoneuroendocrinology 23:219–243, 1998

Simpson E, Pistorello J, Begin A, et al: Use of dialectical behavior therapy in a partial hospital program for women with borderline personality disorder. Psychiatr Serv 49:669–673, 1998

Slawinska U, Kasicki S: Theta-like rhythm in depth EEG activity of hypothalamic areas during spontaneous or electrically induced locomotion in rats. Brain Res 678:117–126, 1995

Smith J: Personality correlates of continuation and outcome in meditation and erect sitting control treatments. J Clin Consult Psychol 46:272–279, 1978

Smith J: Meditation as psychotherapy: a new look at the evidence, in The Psychology of Meditation. Edited by West M. Oxford, England, Clarendon, 1987, pp 136–149

Smith M, Davidson J, Ritchie J, et al: The corticotropin releasing hormone test in patients with posttraumatic stress disorder. Biol Psychiatry 26:349–355, 1989

Smith W, Compton W, West W: Meditation as an adjunct to a happiness enhancement program. J Clin Psychiatry 51:269–273, 1995

Snaith P: Meditation and psychotherapy. Br J Psychiatry 173:193–195, 1998

Sohlberg M, Mateer C: Introduction to Cognitive Rehabilitation. New York, Guilford, 1989

Sommer S, Hassed C: Meditation-based stress management for doctors and students. Med J Aust 163:112, 1995

Spanos N, Stam H, Rivers S, et al: Meditation: expectation and performances on indices of nonanalytic attending. Int J Clin Exp Hypn 28:244–251, 1980

Spencer W, Kandel E: Hippocampal neuron responses to selective activation of recurrent collaterals of hippocampofugal axons. Exp Neurol 4:149–161, 1961

Spiegelman M, Miyuki M: Buddhism and Jungian Psychology. Temple, New Falcon Publications, 1994

Stancak A, Kuna M: EEG changes during forced alternate nostril breathing. Int J Psychophysiol 18:75–79, 1994

Starkman M, Gebarski S, Berent S, et al: Hippocampal formation volume memory dysfunction and cortisol levels in patients with Cushings syndrome. Biol Psychiatry 32:756–765, 1993

Stek R, Bass B: Personal adjustment and perceived locus of control among students interested in meditation. Psychol Rep 32:1019–1022, 1973

Swaab D: Brain aging and Alzheimer's disease: "wear and tear" versus "use it or lose it." Neurobiol Aging 12:317–324, 1991

Sweet M: Enhancing empathy: the interpersonal implications of a Buddhist meditation technique. Psychotherapy 27:19–29, 1990

Taub E, Steiner S, Weingarten E, et al: Effectiveness of broad spectrum approaches to relapse prevention in severe alchoholism: a long-term, randomized, controlled trial of Transcendental Meditation, EMG biofeedback, and electronic neurotherapy. Alcoholism Treatment Quarterly 11:187–220, 1994

Teasdale J, Segal Z, Williams J: How does cognitive therapy prevent depressive relapse and why should attentional control (mindfulness) training help? Behav Res Ther 33:25–39, 1995

Telles S, Naveen K: Yoga for rehabilitation: an overview. Indian J Med Sci 51:123–127, 1997

Thurman R: Tsong Khapa's Speech of Gold in the Essence of True Eloquence: Reason and Enlightenment in the Central Philosophy of Tibet. Princeton, NJ, Princeton University Press, 1984

Thurman R: Essential Tibetan Buddhism. San Francisco, CA, Harper Collins, 1998

Tloczynski J, Tantriella M: A comparison of the effects of Zen breath meditation or relaxation on college adjustment. Psychologia Internationalis: Journal of Psychology of the Orient 41:32–43, 1998

Travis F: The junction-point model: a field model of waking, sleeping, and dreaming, relating dream witnessing, the waking/sleeping transition, and transcendental meditation in terms of a common psychophysiologic state. Dreaming: Journal of the Association for the Study of Dreams 4:91–104, 1994

Turnbull M, Norris H: Effects of transcendental meditation on self-identity indices and personality. Br J Psychol 73:57–68, 1982

Urbanowski F, Miller J: Trauma, psychotherapy, and meditation. Journal of Transpersonal Psychology 28:31–48, 1996

Van Nuys D: Meditation, attention and hypnotic susceptibility: a correlational study. Int J Clin Exp Hypn 21:59–69, 1973

Varela F, Thompson E, Rosch E: The Embodied Mind: Cognitive Science and Human Experience. Cambridge, MA, MIT Press, 1996

Vigne J: Guru and psychotherapist: comparisons from the Hindu tradition. Journal of Transpersonal Psychology 23:121–138, 1991

Wallace A: The Buddhist tradition of Samatha: methods for refining and examining consciousness. Journal of Consciousness Studies 6:175–187, 1999

Wallace R, Benson H, Wilson A: A wakeful hypometabolic physiologic state. Am J Physiol 221:795–799, 1971

Wallace V: Buddhist Tantric medicine in the Kalacakratantra. Journal of the Institute for Buddhist Studies 12:155–174, 1996

Walsh R: Two Asian psychologies and their implications for Western psychotherapists. Am J Psychother 42:543–560, 1988

Walsh R: Meditation research: the state of the art, in Textbook of Transpersonal Psychiatry and Psychology. Edited by Scotten B, Chinnen A, Smith J. New York, Basic Books, 1996

Walsh R, Roche L: Precipitation of acute psychotic episodes by intensive meditation in patients with a history of schizophrenia. Am J Psychiatry 136:1085–1086, 1979

Warrenburg S, Pagano R: Meditation and hemispheric specialization: absorbed attention in long term adherents. Imagination, Cognition, and Personality 2:211–229, 1983

Welwood J: Vulnerability and power in the therapeutic process: existential and Buddhist perspectives. Journal of Transpersonal Psychology 14:118–124, 1982

West M: Traditional and psychological perspectives on meditation, in The Psychology of Meditation. Edited by West M. Oxford, England, Clarendon, 1987, pp 5–22

Wicklund R: Objective self awareness, in Advances in Experimental Social Psychology. Edited by Berkowitz L. New York, Academic, 1975, pp 233–275

Wiesel T, Hubel D: Comparison of the effects of unilateral and bilateral eye closure on cortical unit responses in kittens. J Neurophysiol 28:1029–1040, 1965

Williams R: The Trusting Heart: Great News About Type A Behavior. New York, Random House, 1989

Winterholler M, Erbguth F, Nuendorfer B: Verendung paramedizinischer Verhafen durchMS-Patienten—Patientencharakterisierung und Anwendungswhonheiten. Fortschr Neurol Psychiatr 65:555–561, 1997

Yehuda R: Sensitization of the HPA axis in posttraumatic stress disorder, in Psychobiology of Posttraumatic Stress Disorder. Edited by Yehuda R, MacFarlane A. New York, Academic, 1997, pp 57–75

Zysk K: Asceticism and Healing in Ancient India. Oxford, England, Oxford University Press, 1991

Chapter 5

Complementary Medicine

Implications Toward Medical Treatment and the Patient–Physician Relationship

Catherine C. Crone, M.D.
Thomas N. Wise, M.D.

> It is important to learn not to be angry with opinions different from your own, but to set to work understanding how they came about. If, after you have understood them, they still seem false, you can then combat them more effectually than if you had continued to be merely horrified.
>
> *Bertrand Russell*

Science and technology have benefited patients through the development of more effective medications and other interventions. Patients once faced with limited survival can often look forward to a better prognosis and quality of life. Thus, the increased interest in complementary and alternative medicine (CAM) therapies seems to run counter to the recent advances in modern medicine. Understanding more about the implications behind CAM use is necessary to determine why patients' needs are not satisfied through conventional medicine. For psychiatrists who work with medically ill patients, gaining further knowledge about this trend can be particularly useful. The information obtained can be employed to help patients cope more effectively with their illness and to assist patients in maintaining a constructive relationship with their health care providers.

Definition of Complementary and Alternative Medicine

CAM refers to a broad group of therapeutic approaches that have been difficult to characterize under a single term. Eisenberg et al. (1993) originally defined CAM as medical interventions not widely taught at medical schools or generally available at hospitals in the United States. In recent years, however, the popularity of CAM has risen to the point where some treatments are now offered in hospitals, performed by conventional medical practitioners, and discussed in medical school courses. CAM no longer signifies therapies necessarily outside of allopathic medicine. The present understanding of CAM is best described in Britain and elsewhere as therapies used in conjunction with, rather than instead of, conventional treatments (Cassileth et al. 1996a). This definition, however, still fails to include those who select CAM as a clear alternative to conventional medical care or as a means to prevent illness and bolster general health. Cassileth (1998) has taken these motives into account in her explanation of CAM as *treatments used to promote wellness, those used alongside conventional care, and those used to replace conventional treatments.* One example is the use of herbal medicine, which can be taken to prevent colds, reduce chemotherapy-induced nausea, or combat cancer. Because Cassileth's definition provides a more comprehensive understanding of CAM, we use it in this chapter.

Categories of CAM

Much of the difficulty involved with defining CAM has to do with the large number of practices encompassed within this term. CAM refers to familiar therapies such as hypnosis, acupuncture, meditation, chiropractic, and nutritional supplements. Less popular approaches include energy healing, ayurveda, naturopathy, and Native American practices. Even support groups and psychotherapy/counseling are considered CAM treatments by some authors. Efforts to clarify which practices fall under the title of CAM were started by the National Institutes of Health (NIH) Office of Alternative Medicine (OAM). This agency developed seven major categories for CAM: herbal medicine, mind-body control, pharmacologic or biological treatments, diet/nutrition/lifestyle changes, bioelectromagnetic applications, manual healing, and alternative systems of medical practice (Eskinazi and Hoffman 1998). Table 5–1 list specific CAM treatments within these categories.

General Trends

Studies that have focused on the use of CAM provide evidence of its growing popularity across the United States, the United Kingdom, Canada, and Australia. Surveys among general population samples have suggested lifetime prevalence rates of greater than 60% and annual rates between 15% and 50% (Burg et al. 1998; Eisenberg et al. 1993, 1998; Fulder and Munro 1985; MacLennan et al. 1996; Millar 1997; Thomas et al. 1991). Variability in annual rates is partly a result of whether respondents are asked to consider visits to CAM practitioners only or to include self-administered CAM therapies (e.g., megavitamins, diets). Even more striking are current estimates of the amount of money paid out of pocket for these practices. Based on a recent survey, Eisenberg et al. (1998) estimated that the annual expenditure for CAM in the United States was $27 billion. They felt that this amount was comparable with projected out-of-pocket expenditures for all physician services in the United States. To illustrate this trend further, the authors also found that visits made to CAM practitioners grew from 427 million in 1990 to 629 million by 1997. In addition, demand for herbal medicines and vitamins expanded by 380% and 130%, respectively (Eisenberg et al. 1998).

The increasing appearance of CAM therapies in conventional locations is another indication of their growing popularity. CAM products are now available in local pharmacies, grocery stores, discount warehouse stores, and over the Internet. Many hospitals offer CAM approaches such as massage, acupuncture, and relaxation training as adjuncts to conventional medical interventions. CAM treatments can be obtained in private offices from allopathic physicians and nurses. Publication of specialized telephone directories (e.g., *Alternative Medicine Yellow Pages*) has helped to increase

Table 5–1. Types of complementary and alternative medicine treatments available

Alternative systems of medical practice
Acupuncture
Ayurveda
Homeopathy
Native American practices
Naturopathy
Traditional Oriental medicine

Bioelectromagnetic applications
Electroacupuncture
Electromagnetic fields

Diet/nutrition/lifestyle changes
Fasting
Gerson diet
Livingston-Wheeler diet
Macrobiotic diet
Megavitamins
Nutritional supplements

Herbal medicines
Echinacea
Ginkgo biloba
Ginseng
Hawthorn
Kava kava
St. John's wort

Manual healing
Alexander technique
Chiropractic medicine
Craniosacral therapy
Massage therapy
Osteopathic medicine
Therapeutic touch

Table 5–1.   Types of complementary and alternative medicine treatments available *(continued)*

Mind-body control
  Guided imagery
  Hypnosis
  Meditation
  Prayer
  Qi gong
  Yoga

Pharmacologic and biological treatments
  Antineoplastons
  Cartilage products
  Chelation therapy
  Immunoaugmentative therapy
  Metabolic therapy
  Neural therapy

access to CAM practitioners in the community. Although most CAM services continue to be paid out of pocket, a number of insurance companies provide coverage for certain CAM treatments (e.g., chiropractic, acupuncture) (Moore 1997).

Acceptance of CAM's potential role in medical practice is also reflected in the growth and development of the OAM. Established by Congress in 1992, the office was originally designated the Office of Unconventional Medicine but was later renamed Office of Alternative Medicine (Marwick 1998). It is now called the National Center for Complementary and Alternative Medicine (NCCAM), and its annual funding has recently grown from $20 million to $50 million (Marwick 1998). This new designation coincides with Cassileth's (1998) definition of CAM as both supplemental and alternative to conventional medical care. Thirteen research centers have been funded by the NCCAM that are currently conducting research into the applicability of CAM treatments (Marwick 1998). The NCCAM has also organized multidisciplinary panels that have developed consensus statements about CAM therapies such as acupuncture and behavioral/relaxation techniques (Eskinazi and Hoffman 1998). Development of clinical guidelines is hampered by lack of evidence-based research, and the NCCAM has attempted to address this problem through continued funding and development of studies regarding CAM therapies and specific medical problems. A well-publicized example is the multicenter study of St. John's wort for depression. Additional studies are planned for examining possible benefits of glucosamine for arthritis and acupuncture for depression (Marwick 1998).

CAM Users

Attempts to identify and characterize CAM users demonstrate that a high proportion are Caucasian, female, middle-aged, educated, earn a higher income, and have conventional medicine physicians (Balis et al. 1997; Burg et al. 1998; Eisenberg et al. 1993, 1998; Fulder and Munro 1985; MacLennan et al. 1996; Millar 1997; Thomas et al. 1991). CAM users also tend to seek a more holistic approach to their health and see a mind-body connection to illness and health (Furnham and Bhagrath 1993; Furnham and Forey 1994). The finding that women represent a greater proportion of CAM users is misleading, because they also make up a higher fraction of those using conventional medical care. Women also serve as decision makers regarding the health care needs of other family members.

Additional findings highlight the use of CAM for both preventative and therapeutic aims (Burg et al. 1998; Eisenberg 1993, 1998; Eliason et al. 1997; Fulder and Munro 1985; MacLennan et al. 1996; Millar 1997; Thomas et al. 1991). When chosen for specific therapeutic goals, CAM is often used to treat chronic conditions that do not respond adequately to conventional approaches. Examples include arthritis, back and neck pain, depression, anxiety, colds, allergies, fatigue, and headaches (Burg et al. 1998; Eisenberg 1993, 1998; Fulder and Munro 1985; Jacobs and Crothers 1991; MacLennan et al. 1996; Millar 1997; Paramore 1997; Thomas et al. 1991). CAM is also used in more serious illnesses, as noted by the predominance of inquiries related to cancer that are received by the NCCAM (Marwick 1998). A possible connection between unmet needs from conventional medicine and use of CAM was suggested in the 1994 Robert Wood Johnson Foundation National Access to

Care Survey (Paramore 1997). Findings from additional studies to confirm this finding and to describe these needs in greater detail have yet to be published. Nonetheless, researchers have noted that CAM users often categorize themselves as being in poorer health than those who do not turn to these approaches (Burg et al. 1998; Paramore 1997).

Physicians and CAM

Physicians have traditionally perceived CAM treatments with skepticism and distrust. Lack of sufficient double-blind, placebo-controlled studies is one reason for this viewpoint. Nonetheless, recent surveys suggest that physician attitudes may be changing. Astin et al. (1998) examined surveys from 1982 to 1995 that focused on physician opinions toward five common CAM therapies: massage, chiropractic, acupuncture, herbal medicine, and homeopathy. Approximately half of the physicians surveyed believed in the use of massage, chiropractic, and acupuncture, and a smaller proportion saw a role for the other two approaches. Another survey polled primary care physicians and obstetrics/gynecology clinicians (both physicians and nurse practitioners) working in a large health maintenance organization (HMO) in Northern California and found that most were at least moderately interested in CAM. Among the respondents, over one third of the primary care physicians and nearly half of the obstetrics/gynecology clinicians expressed great interest in CAM. Nearly 90% had recommended some form of CAM therapy to their patients within the past 12 months, even after excluding counseling, special diets, support groups, and religious healing (Gordon et al. 1998). CAM therapies were often suggested for conditions in which the efficacy of conventional treatments was felt to be lacking. A national survey of physicians in family practice, internal medicine, and pediatrics also pointed toward acceptance of several CAM therapies (Berman et al. 1998b). In an examination of physician attitudes toward CAM training, 70% of the family practitioners in the Chesapeake region who responded to a survey wanted training in CAM techniques (Berman et al. 1995). Wetzel and colleagues (1998) found that roughly two-thirds of medical schools in the United States offered electives in CAM or included this topic in required courses. Although physicians may not fully accept CAM, they are recognizing the need to better understand this topic given their influence on patient care.

Whether physicians subscribe to CAM approaches or not, patients do subscribe to them. Because of this, questions have been raised regarding physician responsibility toward their patients with regard to CAM. Attempts to address this issue within the context of medical ethics have been made in studies by Ernst (1997b) and by Sugarman and Burk (1998). Autonomy requires patients to be given an active role in health care decisions but does not require physicians to blindly accept CAM therapies and patients' wishes. Rather, physicians need to be able to share information about treatment options in both conventional medicine and CAM. Patients may be engaged in discussions about CAM or directed to accurate educational resources. Both beneficence and nonmaleficence also apply to considerations about patient care and CAM approaches. They serve as reminders that physicians must focus on the welfare, safety, and well-being of their patients (Ernst 1997b; Sugarman and Burk 1998). Thus, physicians should inquire about CAM therapies and educate patients about those that are safe and effective and those that pose unreasonable risks. The concept of justice refers to patients being provided with reasonable access to treatment options (Sugarman and Burk 1998). This applies to both conventional and CAM approaches. A brief review of the basic concepts in medical ethics may serve to remind physicians that acceptance of CAM is less of a concern compared with the effective handling of this trend and its impact on the on the patient–physician relationship.

CAM and Medical Illness

The application of CAM therapies toward a variety of medical conditions is a common practice (Eisenberg et al. 1993, 1998; Ernst 1998a, 1998c; Ernst and Cassileth 1998; Singh et al. 1996; Snyder 1983). Medically ill patients frequently choose to combine CAM approaches with conventional medical interventions. Studies involving different patient populations indicate that between 24%

and 76% of patients combine these treatments, although many do not tell their physicians about this practice (Cassileth et al. 1984; Drivadhl and Miser 1998; Eisenberg et al. 1993, 1998; Elder et al. 1997; Fulder and Munro 1985; Montbriand 1994; Moser et al. 1996; Thomas et al. 1991). This finding can be significant, because patients are often not aware of the potential complications, drug–drug interactions, and adverse side effects that may appear with these combinations. One problem is that patients do not turn to their health care providers or to licensed CAM practitioners for information. Instead, most use advice provided by family, friends, other patients, media, and the Internet (Crone and Wise 1997; Dimmock et al. 1996; Eliason et al. 1997; Moody et al. 1998). This information varies in quality and may be biased by individual values and commercialism. Concern about this issue was highlighted in a United Kingdom study that found untrained staff at health food stores giving specific treatment advice to an investigator presenting with complaints suggestive of a serious medical condition. Of greatest concern was that few employees recommended the "patient" seek out physician attention (Vickers et al. 1998).

A few research efforts have focused on identifying the underlying factors that contribute to patients' decisions when choosing CAM treatment. Most likely, a number of issues and individual patient characteristics influence this choice (Table 5–2). Chronicity of illness and the experience of being in poorer health appear to contribute to people's desire for CAM, as noted in previous demographic studies (Burg et al. 1998; Eisenberg et al. 1993, 1998; Jacobs and Crothers 1991; Millar 1997; Paramore 1997). Changes in the practice of medical care may be another factor, because financial pressures from reduced reimbursements cause many physicians to limit time spent with patients. This adversely affects the establishment of the traditional patient–physician relationship. In fact, dissatisfaction with conventional medical providers was found to be a major influence in the use of CAM (Furnham and Bhagrath 1993; Furnham and Forey 1994; Sutherland and Verhoef 1994). The nature of a patient's experience with his or her physician does not always predict the decision to use CAM (Astin 1998; Donnelly et al. 1985). Awareness of the risks and

Table 5–2. Possible reasons for using complementary and alternative medicine

Accessibility
Alternative belief system
Adverse reactions from conventional treatments
Distrust of conventional medicine and/or practitioners
Enhancement of general health
Financial concerns
Limitations of conventional treatments
Maintenance of a sense of hope
Management of chronic symptoms
Maximizing treatment options
"Natural" origin
Pressure from family/friends
Preventive measures (e.g., colds, flu, cancer)
Psychologic/coping problems
Sense of control
Side effects from conventional treatments (e.g., nausea, jitteriness)

limitations of conventional interventions may be an additional factor contributing to the demand for CAM approaches. Patients who use homeopathic treatments tend to believe that conventional medicines are ineffective or harmful (Amor and Todd 1985). Acupuncture and homeopathy patients express concern about the potential side effects from conventional treatments (Vincent and Furnham 1996). Homeopathy patients in this group expressed the view that standard therapies were ineffective (Vincent and Furnham 1996). Overt skepticism and criticism toward conventional medicine are contributing factors to CAM use in some of the surveys reviewed (Furnham and Smith 1988; Sutherland and Verhoef 1994).

Attempts to understand CAM use in the context of patient illness behavior have also focused on its possible psychologic benefits. One means by which this has been examined is the concept of internal and external control. In the case of internal control, patients may perceive illness to arise from emotional and lifestyle factors. Thus, treatment of a disease has less to do with the efforts of health care providers and their interventions and more to do with patients' efforts to live a healthy lifestyle and promote feelings of well-being. External control refers to the traditional view that an illness is primarily treated by physicians and their use of conventional approaches. A number of researchers have questioned whether patients turning to CAM are doing so as a means of attaining internal control over their health. Some studies using the Locus of Control Scale have noted that CAM users tend to believe more in internal control and less in the power of their health care providers (Furnham and Forey 1994; Furnham and Smith 1988). Among multiple sclerosis patients, the decision to use CAM was mainly derived from a desire to play an active role in the healing process (Winterholler et al. 1997). This finding was supported in another study by Vincent and Furnham (1996). Although the idea of internal control appears to be connected to CAM and illness behaviors, not all studies have found this to be a motivating factor (Sutherland and Verhoef 1994). An alternative approach has been to consider general views about health and illness. By doing this, researchers have noted that patients using CAM appear to emphasize a more holistic approach to health and perceive illness to be caused by combined internal and external factors (e.g., poor diet, environmental pollution) (Furnham 1994; Furnham and Bhagrath 1993). Present findings support continued study of this concept of internal control and implications toward CAM use. Greater understanding of the influences behind CAM use may allow health care providers to foster a stronger patient–physician relationship and enhance a patients' sense of emotional and physical well being.

Patients who use CAM report more unmet needs for medical care than those who do not, despite more than twice the number of conventional health care visits (Paramore 1997). Although these patients report having more health problems than nonusers, there is the possibility that the unmet needs represent emotional coping difficulties. Whether CAM users have underlying psychiatric pathology and/or coping problems related to their physical health has been considered by only a few researchers. Homeopathy patients showed no differences in psychiatric morbidity compared with those seen in general medical practice (Amor and Todd 1985). A study by Furnham and Bhagrath (1993) compared

80 patients seeing a general practitioner with an equal number attending a homeopath. They found a higher frequency of "minor" (e.g., neurosis) psychiatric problems among the homeopathy patients. Among studies considering the potential contribution of psychologic factors in CAM use, only Davidson and colleagues (1998) examined both personality factors and psychiatric morbidity. Current and lifetime rates of Axis I disorders were recorded by the Structured Clinical Interview for DSM-III-R, whereas personality traits of neuroticism and extraversion were established by the Eysenck Personality Inventory. Patients in both the United States and the United Kingdom participated in this study; those receiving care from CAM practitioners had higher rates of mood and anxiety disorders compared with patient populations receiving conventional medical care. The patients seen by CAM practitioners also tended to be more introverted but not more neurotic (Davidson et al. 1998). These studies present a limited attempt to determine whether undiagnosed and untreated psychologic disorders should be considered when caring for patients using CAM. Further studies may assist physicians in understanding how to better address the gap made by the "unmet needs" in medical care.

CAM and Chronic Illness

Patients contending with chronic illness are often faced with the reality of limited benefits from conventional medical approaches. Although some gain relief from surgery, medicines, dialysis, and physical therapy, others still experience a considerable number of symptoms because of poor response to these treatments. Under these circumstances, physicians are not surprised that patients might abandon conventional medicine. However, most patients who select CAM therapies do not stop seeing their physicians or using prescribed interventions. Instead, they combine the approaches in hopes of achieving the best outcome possible. Physicians caring for those with chronic illness may want to be aware of particular CAM treatments their patients might use. This can help to guide discussions about CAM and encourage learning more about potential benefits and risks of specific therapies. The primary goal would be to optimize patient care through prudent use of CAM and conventional treatments while avoiding any unnecessary risks. The following section discusses the common CAM approaches that dominate certain patient populations with chronic illness.

Arthritis, Low Back Pain, and Fibromyalgia

Rheumatologic disorders are often difficult to treat because of their limited response to medicines and other interventions. Even when interventions do prove useful, there is a significant risk of adverse side effects and complications. Potential problems include steroid-induced diabetes and mood changes, ulcers and hemorrhage related to use of nonsteroidal anti-inflammatory drugs (NSAIDs), and infections caused by surgical procedures.

Emotional distress from chronic pain, fatigue, and disability is another obstacle to treatment. General surveys of patients in rheumatology clinics reveal rates of CAM use ranging from 30% to nearly 100% (Boisset and Fitzcharles 1994; Cronan et al. 1989; Kronenfeld and Wasner 1982; Resch et al. 1997; Vecchio 1994). Manual therapies, including acupuncture, chiropractic, and massage, are popular choices that require visits to CAM practitioners. Most patients perceive only moderate benefits from these treatments (Resch et al. 1997). Although arthritis patients report a greater benefit from conventional therapies, visits to CAM practitioners are rated as much more satisfying than those with general practitioners (Ernst 1998c). This effect may be the result of CAM practitioners spending time with patients, the practitioners' added focus on emotional and lifestyle factors, their empathic listening, and their physical connection with patients (e.g., through chiropractic, massage, touch therapies). Patients with arthritis frequently use self-administered approaches such as prayer, exercise, diet, and vitamins (Boisset and Fitzcharles 1994; Cronan et al. 1989; Kronenfeld and Wasner 1982). Although an OAM consensus panel found considerable evidence supporting use of relaxation techniques for management of chronic pain, only one study mentions the use of relaxation techniques by a patient population surveyed (Eskinazi and Hoffman 1998).

Fibromyalgia is a rheumatologic condition affecting younger patients that causes considerable loss of functioning and reduced quality of life. Management of the pain and fatigue that characterize this disorder is complicated because they are often resistant to conventional treatments. This difficulty may account for the particularly high rate of CAM use in this group, which ranges from 70% to almost 100% (Dimmock et al. 1996; Nicassio et al. 1997; Pioro-Boisset et al. 1996). Those suffering for longer periods of time, experiencing greater pain, and having higher disability turned to a broad range of CAM approaches (Dimmock et al. 1996; Fitzcharles and Esdaile 1997; Nicassio et al. 1997). Many chose to combine self-administered therapy with those that were practitioner provided (e.g., acupuncture, osteopathy) (Dimmock et al. 1996). The self-administered treatments appeared to be more popular, and mainly consisted of diets, herbal medicine, vitamins/minerals, and fish oils (Dimmock et al. 1996; Nicassio et al. 1997; Pioro-Boisset et al. 1996). Use of prayer/spirituality was also common and may reflect a need for hope and emotional support while living with an ill-defined, treatment-resistant illness (Nicassio et al. 1997; Pioro-Boisset et al. 1996).

Chiropractic

Chiropractic is one of the most popular CAM approaches. It also has wide acceptance among conventional medical practitioners. Based on the premise that manipulation of the vertebrae corrects misalignments of the spine (subluxation) and allows the body to heal itself, chiropractic is licensed in all 50 states and currently administered by 50,000 providers (Kaptchuk and Eisenberg 1998). A majority of states has mandated health insurance coverage for these treatments, which are primarily sought out for low back pain (Kaptchuk and Eisenberg 1998). The Agency for Health Care Policy and Research (AHCPR), after completing an extensive review of literature in 1994, supported the efficacy of chiropractic for acute low back pain (Berman et al. 1998a). However, no conclusions could be reached for its use in chronic low back pain.

Studies that compare chiropractic with conventional management of low back pain tend to show some benefits from chiropractic (Cherkin et al. 1998), and meta-analyses of various studies involving chiropractic treatment also tend to justify its role in acute low back pain (R. Anderson et al. 1992; Shekelle et al. 1992). Despite this, there is an overall lack of studies of adequate quality and methodology. Evidence supporting the benefit of chiropractic in other conditions, such as neck pain, headache, and asthma, is also inadequate (Kaptchuk and Eisenberg 1998). Adverse effects of chiropractic are not infrequent, although most are considered mild and transient (e.g., local or radiating discomfort, headache, fatigue) (Senstad et al. 1996, 1997). In a small number of cases, manipulation of the lower spine can result in cauda equina syndrome (Kaptchuk and Eisenberg 1998). Cervical adjustments are linked to a greater number of serious complications, such as disc injury, vertebrobasilar infarction, vertebral fracture, carotid hematoma, and Wallenberg's syndrome (Alimi et al. 1996a, 1996b; Kaptchuk and Eisenberg 1998; Klougart et al. 1996; Studdert et al. 1998). Risks from chiropractic manipulation are greatest in certain conditions (e.g., osteoporosis, spinal cord or nerve root compression, severe degenerative changes or long-standing spinal deformity, recent whiplash injury, vertebrobasilar insufficiency), and this procedure should therefore be avoided in patients with these conditions (Berman et al. 1998a).

Acupuncture

Acupuncture is another CAM technique gaining popularity among conventional health care providers. The NIH Consensus Statement on Acupuncture (1998) indicates that there is evidence for its use in postoperative and chemotherapy-induced nausea and vomiting, postoperative pain, low back pain, and myofascial pain. Clinical trials also suggest benefits in fibromyalgia, osteoarthritis, menstrual cramps, headaches, stroke rehabilitation, and addictions (National Institutes of Health Consensus Panel 1998). Adequate numbers of high-quality, methodologically sound studies for these latter conditions are generally lacking (Berman et al. 1999; National Institutes of Health Consensus Panel 1998). One high-quality study compared fibromyalgia patients receiving real acupuncture with those given sham treatment (i.e., superficial needle placement in a nonacupuncture point). Those in the real acupuncture group exhibited significantly more improvement in their fibromyalgia symptoms compared with those in the sham group as rated by both patients and physicians. However, some patients receiving real acupuncture experienced worsening of their fibromyalgia pain (Berman et al. 1999).

The analgesic effects of acupuncture appear to result from changes produced in the spinal cord and brain (National Institutes of Health Consensus Panel 1998). Endogenous opioids are released peripherally and neurotransmitters and hormones (e.g., adrenocorticotropic hormone) are released centrally (Cencieros and Brown 1998; National Institutes of Health Consensus Panel 1998). Complications from acupuncture treatments are rare, although cases of hepatitis, pneumothorax, HIV, endocarditis, and other problems have been reported (Ernst 1997a). These problems can be minimized by proper needle use (see Chapter 2 by Rainone, this volume). Berman et al. (1998b) advise against acupuncture for pregnant patients and those with bleeding disorders, cardiac valve disease, and skin infections; patients with pacemakers, cardiac arrhythmias, or epilepsy should avoid electroacupuncture. To ensure safety and adequate quality, there have been attempts to standardize training programs and require credentialing and licensure for acupuncture providers (National Institutes of Health Consensus Panel 1998).

Inflammatory Bowel Disease

Inflammatory bowel disease (IBD), which includes Crohn's disease and ulcerative colitis, tends to affect young adult patients and result in chronic problems marked by repeated remissions and exacerbations. Patients may undergo surgical interventions and take immunosuppressive agents that cause marked changes in body image (e.g., ostomy). This often occurs during an important phase of adult development when patients are beginning to date, marry, raise children, and start careers. Coping with these challenges in the midst of chronic illness can become overwhelming. Among studies of CAM use in IBD patients, Moser et al. (1996) noted that those with longer illness duration, greater concerns about surgery, and fears of feeling out of control or of being treated as different were more likely to turn to CAM approaches. The impact of repeated life disruptions caused by IBD was also evident in study of more than 200 IBD patients by Hilsden et al. (1998b). Both disease duration and a history of hospitalizations were the strongest predictors of CAM use in this group. Regaining a sense of control over one's health was another theme contributing to interest in CAM, as cited by Verhoef et al. (1998) and Hilsden et al. (1998b). Limited therapeutic benefits, along with disagreeable side effects from conventional treatments, were added factors that influenced the use of CAM therapies (Verhoef et al. 1998). Patients incorporating CAM approaches tended to select oral agents, especially homeopathic and herbal medicines (Hilsden et al. 1998b; Moody et al. 1998; Verhoef et al. 1998; Verhoef and Sutherland 1990). Other popular treatments included dietary manipulation, vitamins, naturopathy, and mind-body techniques. Lack of knowledge and understanding about IBD was not a factor in the use of CAM, because those who felt well informed about the illness still wanted education about CAM practices (Hilsden et al. 1998a).

Renal Failure

Management of renal disease through the use of herbal medicine has been practiced since Roman times and was recorded by Pliny the Elder (Aliotta and Pollio 1994; De Matteis Tortora 1994). Disorders that produce acute or chronic renal failure lead to a variety of troubling signs and symptoms. Anemia, hypertension, malaise, peripheral edema, osteodystrophy, pruritus, and uremia-induced cognitive and mood disturbances commonly occur. Management of renal failure requires dialysis treatments that are lengthy, uncomfortable, and often leave patients feeling fatigued and unwell. Accompanying dietary restrictions, fluid limits, and multiple medications add to the patient's burden. In light of these requirements, CAM use is not surprising. Few studies have examined this issue in renal patients, although Snyder (1983) found that 74% of adult hemodialysis patients ($n = 230$) acknowledged trying one or more CAM practices. Prayer or faith healing, exercise, herbal medicine, and massage were desirable choices, with most patients feeling some benefit from their practices. Patients turned to CAM mainly for relief from physical symptoms linked to renal failure and dialysis, for enhancement of emotional well-being, and for improvement of kidney function (Snyder 1983). This last reason was also a motivating force among patients seen at a transplant center who responded to a questionnaire regarding the use of herbal medicines and nutritional supplements (Crone and Wise 1997). Despite the wish for herbal medicines that might preserve renal functioning, there are numerous reports of renal impairment from toxic botanical agents (Foote and Cohen 1998). A recent string of cases involving renal failure in young women was found to be caused by the substitution of a nephrotoxic herb for a benign herb in a natural weight-loss regimen (But 1993; Depierreuz et al. 1994; van Ypersele and Vanherweghem 1995; Vanhaelen et al. 1994; Vanherweghem et al. 1993).

Dementia

Advertisements for products aimed at boosting alertness and cognitive functioning appear in magazines, newspapers, television, and radio. In modern society, having the ability to manage one's affairs independently is valued, whereas impairment from Alzheimer's disease or other forms of dementia is greatly feared. A small number of studies have questioned caregivers of dementia patients about the use of CAM therapies for memory enhancement. Only a 10% rate of CAM use was discovered in a Canadian study, but a North Carolina survey found that more than one-half of family caregivers had tried at least one type of CAM practice on their relative with Alzheimer's disease (Coleman et al. 1995; Hogan and Ebly 1996). Both studies showed that vitamins/minerals, herbal medicines, and health foods were used most often. In the American survey, most caregivers did not observe significant memory improvement despite addition of CAM treatments early in the course of the Alzheimer's disease (Coleman et al. 1995). One-quarter of the caregivers also experimented with CAM to help control problematic behaviors resulting from dementia (Coleman et al. 1995). However, only one-third of these felt there was any beneficial response. Notably, the level of caregiver frustration and the presence of problem behaviors did not influence the decision to use CAM practices (Coleman et al. 1995).

Herbal Medicine

Knowledge of the medicinal properties of certain plants has been in existence for centuries and used in the treatment of various conditions. Modern technology has allowed these plants to be studied further, facilitating the identification and isolation of active pharmacologic compounds; this has resulted in the manufacture of conventional drugs containing chemicals originally derived from herbal remedies (e.g., digoxin, warfarin, ephedrine). Thus, the concept of deriving therapeutic benefits from herbal medicines is based on scientific fact. Demand for this form of CAM has grown rapidly within the past few years, creating a multibillion-dollar industry (Eisenberg et al. 1998). The problem that exists for most herbal medicines, however, is a lack of scientific studies establishing the presence of pharmacologic activity and safety. Current regulations do not require these agents to undergo the scrutiny required for prescription drugs, and loopholes permit herbal medicines to be sold without assurances of safety, purity, and efficacy (Crone and Wise 1998). Specific problems have arisen from the substitution of one herbal ingredient for another in a commercial product. This can be caused by accidental misidentification of a plant or intentional substitution of an herb for one that is cheaper or more readily available (Crone and Wise 1998). Unlabeled substitution has resulted in cases of renal failure, anticholinergic delirium, and hepatic impairment (Crone and Wise 1998; Ernst 1998b). Adulteration of an herbal medicine with conventional drugs (e.g., steroids, benzodiazepines, NSAIDs) and heavy metals has also occurred, leading to unexpected complications (Crone and Wise 1998; Ernst 1998b). Although many plants do contain pharmacologic agents, a number also include compounds that can be toxic to humans (Table 5–3). Concern about toxicity is especially high for pregnant women, children, and elderly patients and for those who are medically ill (Crone and Wise 1998). Another consideration is the limited understanding among both patients and practitioners of the risk for drug–drug interactions (Table 5–4) (Crone and Wise 1998; Ernst 1998b; L. G. Miller 1998). Part of the problem comes from the presence of multiple chemical compounds in a single plant, making attempts to isolate and identify all active ingredients a complicated task.

Table 5–3. Potential toxicity and adverse reactions from herbal medicines

Common name	Botanical name	Purported use	Potential toxicity
Aloe	*Aloe vera*	Wound healing Health tonic	Dehydration, diarrhea Nausea/vomiting
Black cohosh	*Cimicifuga racemosa*	Arthritis Premenstrual syndrome	Nausea/vomiting Uterine contractions
Chaparral	*Larrea tridentata*	Anticancer Antioxidant Arthritis	Hepatotoxic
Comfrey	*Symphytum officinale*	Digestive aid Wound healing	Hepatotoxic
Ginseng	*Panax ginseng*	Adaptogen Aphrodisiac Stimulant	Hypertension, anxiety Depression, agitation Mastalgia, insomnia
Hawthorn	*Crataegeus laevigata* *Crataegeus monogyna*	Angina Congestive heart failure	Hypotension
Kava kava	*Piper methysticum*	Anxiolytic Sedative	Dermatitis, dyspnea Hallucinations
Licorice	*Glycyrrhiza glabra*	Arthritis Improves liver function Antiulcer agent	Arrhythmia, edema Hypokalemia, hypertension

Table 5–3. Potential toxicity and adverse reactions from herbal medicines *(continued)*

Common name	Botanical name	Purported use	Potential toxicity
Ma huang	*Ephedra sinica*	Antiasthmatic Stimulant	Hypertension, anxiety Tachycardia, mania
Mistletoe	*Viscum album*	Anticancer Antihypertensive Immunostimulant	Bradycardia, delirium Nausea, hypertension Gastroenteritis
Pau d'arco	*Tabebuia impetiginosa* *Tabebuia avellanedae*	Anticancer Immunostimulant	Nausea/vomiting Anemia, hemorrhage
Poke root	*Phytolacca americana*	Arthritis Rheumatism	Hepatotoxic

Table 5–4. Potential drug–drug interactions with herbal medicines

Potential interaction	Herbal medicine	Prescription or over-the-counter drug
Anticholinergic delirium	Burdock[a] Lobelia Thornapple Skullcap	Antihistamines Antispasmodic agents Antiparkinsonian agents Antipsychotic agents Tricyclic antidepressants
Cardiac arrhythmia (digitalis toxicity)	Foxglove Hawthorn Lily-of-the-valley Squill	Digoxin
Hemorrhage	Dong quai Feverfew Garlic Ginger Ginkgo Ginseng Chamomile	Heparin Warfarin Nonsteroidal anti-inflammatory drugs Platelet aggregation inhibitors
Hypoglycemia	Bitter melon Fenugreek Garlic Ginger Ginseng *Gymnema sylvestre*	Insulin Oral antihyperglycemic agents
Hypokalemia	Aloe Buckthorn Dandelion Juniper Licorice	Diuretic agents
Hypotension	Hawthorn	Antihypertensive agents
Oversedation	Catnip Hops Kava kava Passion flower Valerian	Barbiturates Benzodiazepines Hypnotic agents (e.g., zolpidem) Opiates

[a]Contamination with belladonna is common.

CAM and Life-Threatening Illness

Life-threatening disorders such as cancer, HIV, and asthma can appear as either acute or chronic threats to bodily integrity and patient survival. For some, these illnesses produce a rapid decline in health with subsequent mortality, whereas others experience recurrent episodes of remission and relapse, requiring repeated hospitalizations. Although advances in conventional medicine have been helpful (e.g., protease inhibitors in AIDS), many therapies yield only temporary control of a disease. Those seeking to maximize their chance of survival, quality of life, or sense of control may incorporate CAM approaches into their medical regimens. Observations made in these patient groups reveal a high rate of CAM use and growing demand for information on their potential therapeutic benefits. In the following section, this phenomenon is discussed in greater detail.

Asthma

Most asthma patients must cope with a chronic and recurring illness that poses a considerable threat to daily functioning. More than 12 million Americans have asthma, and asthma causes over 100 million patient-days of restricted activity annually (Hackman et al. 1996). In the past two decades, there has been a marked rise in the number of patients diagnosed with this disease along with sharp increases in the number of hospitalizations and deaths (Hackman et al. 1996). Theophylline, bronchodilators, or corticosteroids help to reduce symptoms caused by bronchoconstriction and excess mucus formation, but they tend to produce unwanted side effects (e.g., tremor, anxiety, cushingoid changes). A desire to control asthma beyond conventional means has been observed by those studying this population (Blanc et al. 1997; Ernst 1998a, 1998d, 1999). Herbal medicines, caffeinated beverages, relaxation techniques, dietary supplements, homeopathy, and acupuncture have been tried by adults and children. Recent surveys by Ernst (1998a, 1998d) revealed that nearly 60% of adult asthma patients had experience with CAM, and one-third of children with the disorder had been administered these therapies. Notably, more than 70% of the parents of asthmatic children were willing to consider

CAM approaches (Ernst 1998d). For the adult group, severity of asthma was linked to use of more types of CAM (Ernst 1998a).

Several reviews have examined the evidence for CAM in asthma, but conclusions remain limited because of study size and methodology (But and Chang 1996; Davis et al. 1998; Lewith 1998; Lewith and Watkins 1996; Vickers and Smith 1997). Chinese herbal medicines show therapeutic activity from the sympathomimetic agents (e.g., ma huang, pinella) incorporated into them (But and Chang 1996; Hackman et al. 1996). Other herbs have mucolytic, cough suppressant, or cromolyn sodium–type effects (But and Chang 1996; Hackman et al. 1996). Not all herbs have effects that are beneficial, however, and several have led to reports of serious adverse reactions (Crone and Wise 1998). Homeopathy is a another popular choice, although investigators have failed to find evidence supporting its function in treating asthma (Ernst 1999; Lewith and Watkins 1996). Vitamins B and C, along with magnesium, also have been studied, but results are conflicting (Lewith 1998; Lewith and Watkins 1996).

Relaxation techniques and acupuncture have been studied more thoroughly, and the results are suggestive of a benefit to patients (Davis et al. 1998; National Institutes of Health Consensus Panel 1998; Lewith and Watkins 1996; Vickers and Smith 1997). One well-organized study compared patients who were taught to perform daily yoga and meditation with patients in a control group. Significant reductions in the number of asthma attacks and use of medications along with improvement in peak expiratory flow were observed (Nagarathna and Nagendra 1985). Although Ernst (1999) and Davis et al. (1998) reviewed acupuncture studies separately and failed to find adequate proof of effectiveness, the NIH Consensus Panel's (1998) review did find clinical evidence supporting an adjunctive role for this treatment.

Homeopathy

Homeopathic medicine is based on the idea that highly dilute substances possess therapeutic benefit. Derived from plants, minerals, animal products, or chemicals, selected agents must be able to produce symptoms similar to those being experienced by the patient (Cassileth 1998). Remedies are believed to become more potent as they undergo repeated dilution and agitation, resulting in a solution with trace amounts of the original substance (Cassileth 1998). Resurgence in interest in homeopathic medicine has been recognized in the United States and the United Kingdom, where homeopathic agents are often used for prevention and treatment of self-limiting disorders (e.g., colds, flu, allergies) (Ernst 1996; Jacobs and Crothers 1991). Some patients select them for management of chronic and life-threatening illnesses (e.g., asthma, IBD) (Ernst 1998d, 1999; Moser et al. 1996; Verhoef et al. 1998). This current popularity confounds conventional practitioners, who often perceive homeopathic agents as simple placebos. Numerous studies of homeopathy in the treatment of medical conditions exist, and some authors have tried to review them. Kleijnen et al. (1991) systematically examined 107 controlled trials; many of the studies demonstrated positive results beyond those expected. No conclusions could be reached in this review because of limitations in the quality and design of these studies. Linde and colleagues (1997) reviewed placebo-controlled trials, including current studies of the therapeutic effects of homeopathy. Their meta-analysis revealed that clinical response was not fully due to placebo. Although these results were suggestive, the overall evidence failed to establish the clinical effectiveness of homeopathy for any isolated condition. Determining the true reason for positive response remains a question needing further study. Patients interested in homeopathy should be aware that practitioners vary in the extent of therapeutic claims made, and that no licensure requirements exist in most states (Studdert et al. 1998).

HIV Disease

Most of the studies regarding CAM use among HIV-positive patients were performed before the current boom in combination therapy with protease inhibitors and antiretroviral agents. For many, this has led to control of viral replication and complications to the point of restoring life expectancy and functional capacity. Despite these advances, there are patients who do not respond to these drugs. In addition, both medications produce a number of problematic side effects, including nausea, vomiting, diarrhea, fatigue, headache, and hematologic alterations. The gastrointestinal side effects are particularly troubling, as many patients struggle to maintain adequate nutritional status, body weight, and muscle mass (Elion and Cohen 1997). Rates of CAM use have been found to range from about one-third to more than two-thirds of the populations surveyed (W. Anderson et al. 1993; Barton et al. 1989; Fairfield et al. 1998; Hand 1989; Kassler and Blanc 1991; Langewitz and Ruttimann 1994; Ostrow et al. 1997; Singh et al. 1996). Most patients perceived benefits from CAM treatments that were mainly chosen to enhance immune function, fight infections, treat pain, prevent weight loss, manage gastrointestinal symptoms, or reduce stress (Barton et al. 1989; Fairfield et al. 1998; Langewitz and Ruttimann 1994; Ostrow et al. 1997). Both nutritional supplements and herbal medicines were prevailing choices, although acupuncture, massage, and other mind-body therapies also were selected (W. Anderson et al. 1993; Barton et al. 1989; Fairfield et al. 1998; Hand 1989; Kassler and Blanc 1991; Langewitz and Ruttimann 1994; Ostrow et al. 1997; Singh et al. 1996). Notably, one study that inquired about the use of herbal medicines discovered patients who were taking them while simultaneously enrolled in clinical drug trials (Kassler and Blanc 1991). Whether these herbals interacted with the study drugs was unknown.

Attempts to characterize patients who are prone to select CAM therapies have yielded conflicting results. Although some researchers have noted a connection to greater levels of emotional distress, higher income or education, and duration of seropositivity, others have failed to achieve similar results (W. Anderson et al. 1993; Langewitz and Ruttimann 1994; Ostrow et al. 1997). An important finding by Langewitz and Ruttimann (1994), who observed higher levels of depression and anxiety among those using CAM, was that these patients had realistic expectations about the course of their illness. A study by Singh and colleagues (1996) suggests that patients who use CAM therapies may be less discouraged and more hopeful about their condition than those who do not.

Nutritional Supplements

Public interest in the use of antioxidant vitamins (i.e., vitamins A, C, E, beta-carotene) to reduce the risk of developing cancer and cardiovascular disease has been one reason behind the current demand for nutritional supplements (Reynolds 1994). Epidemiologic and scientific studies have tended to support the role of supplements in preventive health, although some results have been conflicting (Garewal and Diplock 1995; Halbert 1997; Herbert 1994; Hunt 1996; Meyers et al. 1996; Reynolds 1994). Recognition of the negative effects of osteoporosis on quality of life has led to a market for calcium supplements among pre- and postmenopausal women. Zinc, selenium, and chromium picolinate are other popular items chosen for a variety of potential benefits, including weight loss, antioxidant effects, better control of diabetic blood sugar levels, and immune system enhancement (Beltz and Doering 1993; Halbert 1997). For certain patient groups, the need for supplementation is evident because of higher incidences of anorexia, cachexia, and vitamin deficiency (e.g., cancer, diabetes, HIV, elderly) (Elion and Cohen 1997; Hunt 1996). Appropriate supplementation can boost chances of patient survival and improve daily functioning (Elion and Cohen 1997). Concerns about patient health and the use of vitamins/minerals occur in the practice of megavitamin therapy. When taken in large doses, some supplements can produce toxic reactions (Bendich 1992; G. R. Brown and Greenwood 1987; DiPalma and Ritchie 1977; Flodin 1990; Meyers et al. 1996). Patients with renal or hepatic impairment, poor nutritional status, or coagulation disorders are more prone to adverse effects from this approach (Table 5–5) (Meyers et al. 1996).

Hormonal supplements have also received much attention, especially dehydroepiandrosterone (DHEA). Secreted by adrenal glands and converted into testosterone and estrogen, DHEA has been purported to have antiaging and cancer-protective effects. Studies have yielded mixed results, with some suggesting that higher DHEA levels increase the risk for hormone-sensitive cancers (i.e., breast, prostate, ovarian) (Paulsen 1998). Other supplements have become prevalent only in certain patient groups, such as shark cartilage among cancer patients, which is based on the idea that shark cartilage interferes with tumor vascularization. However, this claim has not been supported by subsequent research (Cassileth 1999; Cassileth and Chapman 1996b; D. R. Miller

Table 5–5. Potential toxicity and adverse reactions from nutritional supplements

Supplement	Dose	Duration	Potential toxicity
Vitamin A	500,000 IU 100,000 IU/day	Single dose Months/years	Somnolence Fatigue Headache Anorexia Bone/joint pain Hepatomegaly Hypercalcemia
Vitamin D	≥40,000 IU/day	Months/years	Nausea/vomiting Headache Weight loss Apathy Fatigue Confusion Renal impairment Osteoporosis
Vitamin C	>3 g/day	Days/years	Diarrhea Kidney stones Impaired iron absorption Coagulopathy[a]

Table 5–5. Potential toxicity and adverse reactions from nutritional supplements *(continued)*

Supplement	Dose	Duration	Potential toxicity
Vitamin B_6	> 50 mg/day	Months	Convulsions Headache Fatigue Ataxia Peripheral neuropathy
Chromium picolinate	Unknown	Unknown	Hypoglycemia
DHEA	Unknown	Unknown	Increased risk of ovarian, breast, prostate cancer
Melatonin	> 1 mg hs	Days/months	Fatigue Dizziness Headache Irritability Abdominal cramps
Niacin	> 300 mg/day > 2.5 g/day	Single dose–months Months	Nausea Diarrhea Flushing Abnormal liver enzymes Hyperglycemia
Shark cartilage	60–80 mg/day	Unknown	One case of reversible hepatotoxicity

Note. DHEA = dehydroepiandrosterone.
[a]Reduces prothrombin time in patients receiving warfarin or heparin.

et al. 1998; Paulsen 1998). Another popular item is glucosamine for patients with arthritis. Readily available in stores, this product is scheduled for further study through support from the NCCAM (Eskinazi and Hoffman 1998). As new products continue to appear, patients and caregivers should know that research establishing safety and therapeutic efficacy will lag behind efforts aimed at marketing and availability.

Cancer

Despite advances in the early detection and treatment of cancer, this illness remains a significant source of fear and trepidation. In recent years, there has been strong interest in potential benefits offered by CAM treatments toward the prevention, treatment, and management of cancer and its related side effects (e.g., chemotherapy-induced nausea, fatigue). This trend is noted by the NCCAM, which has received a majority of inquiries related to cancer (Marwick 1998). Acknowledgment from government agencies and cancer researchers has led to the development of a formal collaboration between the NCCAM and the National Cancer Institute (NCI) and to the formation of an advisory panel to guide research efforts regarding CAM use in the treatment of cancer (Marwick 1998). A large number of studies have reported on the prevalence of CAM use among cancer patients, which ranges from 16% to 91% (Cassileth et al. 1984; Crocetti et al. 1998; Elder et al. 1997; Liu et al. 1997; Munsted et al. 1996; Oneschuk et al. 1998; Risberg et al. 1997, 1998a; VandeCreek et al. 1999). Ernst and Cassileth (1998) reviewed 26 studies and found an average prevalence rate of about 31%. Studies attempting to identify the patients most likely to use CAM have tried to determine whether there are connections with cancer type, duration, or diagnostic staging. Results have been mixed, although patients with metastatic disease are generally more willing to try radical CAM treatments (e.g., metabolic therapy, antineoplastons) (Ernst and Cassileth 1998). Other factors that might influence the decision about CAM have been examined, and beliefs concerning cancer etiology play a contributing role. Three studies connect CAM use to patients' belief that cancer onset was caused by psychologic distress (P. J. Brown and Carney 1996; Cassileth et al. 1984; Munsted et al. 1996). An additional influence was cited by some patients who turned to CAM seeking relief from coping problems and wanting a sense of control (Crocetti et al. 1998; Davidson et al. 1998; Ernst and Cassileth 1998; Munsted et al. 1996; Risberg et al. 1998a). Additional motivating factors were the desire to boost the immune system's ability to fight cancer, to enhance the effects of conventional treatments, to prevent disease recurrence or progression, and to directly cure cancer (Davidson et al. 1998; Liu et al. 1997; Munsted et al. 1996; Risberg et al. 1998b).

Cassileth noted that cancer patients use CAM therapies as alternatives to conventional approaches (i.e., radiation, chemotherapy, surgery) or as adjunctive agents to promote general well-being and control of undesirable symptoms (Cassileth 1999; Cassileth and Chapman 1996a, 1996b). Different types of CAM have been popular, although those used as alternative cancer interventions have not been supported by results from subsequent research. Among these choices are metabolic therapies, essiac, iscador, megavitamins, macrobiotic diet, shark cartilage, antineoplastons, and immunoaugmentative therapy. Metabolic therapies are based on the idea that toxic agents from cancer cells collect in the liver, leading to organ failure and death (Cassileth 1999). To counteract this, patients follow a low-salt, low-fat, and high-potassium diet and undergo coffee enemas (Cassileth 1999). Both essiac and iscador are herbal medicines whose efficacy has not been established (Cassileth and Chapman 1996a, 1996b; Kaegi 1998a, 1998b). Iscador is an extract of European mistletoe, which can produce nausea, bradycardia, delirium, and elevated blood pressure (Paulsen 1998). Both of these products are banned in the United States but can be obtained in neighboring countries. Antineoplastons are peptides originally isolated from human urine and are promoted by a clinic in Texas (Cassileth and Chapman 1996a, 1996b). Research performed by the NCI and in Canada failed to demonstrate benefits from this treatment (Cassileth 1999).

Although CAM therapies have not been effective as alternatives to conventional treatment, they may provide assistance as adjunctive agents. Relaxation techniques such as meditation, hypnosis, and yoga can be effective for coping with stress and managing nausea or discomfort (Cassileth 1999; Eskinazi and Hoffman

1998). Massage and therapeutic touch can be used for similar purposes, and they have no risks of adverse effects (Cassileth 1999). Herbal teas brewed from ginger, chamomile, and peppermint reduce chemotherapy-induced nausea. However, patients with coagulation disorders or taking blood thinners may experience worsening of the coagulation disorder or an intensified anticoagulant effect from chamomile or ginger (Cassileth 1999; Crone and Wise 1998). Valerian and kava kava possess sedative and hypnotic activity, but their safety and efficacy have not been proven (Crone and Wise 1998). Future research about CAM and cancer management should help guide health care providers in discussing and recommending approaches most likely to benefit their patients.

CAM and the Patient–Physician Relationship

Given the continued demand for CAM therapies, physicians are faced with deciding how to handle this phenomenon among their patients. The classic parental relationship between patient and physician has been in a state of evolution for some time, even before the rise in CAM use. Patients no longer simply accept diagnoses and follow treatments with minimal questioning, nor should they. Instead, they often do their own research into treatment options while learning about them from their health care providers. Many patients become quite knowledgeable about risks and benefits (e.g., side effects, complications, response rates, quality of life) offered by conventional medical therapy. A desire for a more active role in making treatment decisions has led to the need for alterations in patient–physician communication. Providing time for questions, second opinions, and added sources for information can serve to strengthen the alliance between patient and provider. This change in dialogue is also necessary with CAM approaches to strengthen the patient–physician relationship.

The importance of developing a dialogue with patients who are interested in or are already using CAM approaches is evident in several of the studies included in this chapter. Eisenberg and colleagues (1993, 1998) reported that most patients fail to inform their health care providers about their CAM therapies. This lack of communication exists despite the possibility of adverse side effects, complications, and drug–drug interactions. Patients may unknowingly harm themselves or alter the effectiveness of their conventional treatments. Even when patients do experience problems with CAM, they appear to have a higher threshold for reporting them compared with those arising from prescribed approaches (Barnes et al. 1998). In addition, some patients describe an unwillingness to discuss CAM with their physicians because of concerns about being "scorned" or criticized (VandeCreek et al. 1999). Regardless of whether there is a basis for them, these perceptions threaten to harm the therapeutic alliance and related patient care. A number of studies also note that patients refrained from raising this topic because they believed their physicians to be poorly informed, disinterested, or avoidant regarding CAM treatments (Gray et al. 1998; Verhoef et al. 1998). Indeed, some doctors have expressed highly negative views of CAM in journal commentaries. Other physicians place the responsibility of discussing this issue on their patients (Gray et al. 1998). Clearly, this standoff does not serve either party. Patients not only need examinations, tests, and procedures, but they also want assistance in the task of coping with their illnesses. If they fail to receive this support from their physicians, some will turn to CAM approaches and practitioners in hopes of meeting these needs. For psychiatrists working with the medically ill, awareness of these issues allows them to help other physicians in understanding their patients' concerns. Psychiatrists will also be better equipped to support patients faced with a loss of control, declining health, and an unknown future.

What can physicians do to broach the topic of CAM and maintain their therapeutic alliance with patients? The first step requires incorporating questions about CAM into regular history-taking (Lazar and O'Connor 1998). By doing this, patients experience less trepidation about raising the topic and may perceive their physicians as being willing to discuss this issue further. In fact, patients have expressed a desire for information and advice about CAM therapies from their health care providers (Gray et al. 1998). Doctors must recall that use of CAM does not represent a wish to undermine conventional care. Rather, most patients are simply looking to enhance general health, emotional well-being, and effects of their prescribed treatments while also managing unwanted side effects and symptoms. Most patients are unaware of the potential risks posed by CAM therapies and appreciate the knowledge shared. Physicians can help patients to weigh the risks and benefits of these treatment modes, much as they already do with conventional approaches. Patients can be advised about CAM therapies that may offer more benefits and less risk of harm. Even when physicians are unable to give much information to their patients, their discussion of CAM affords the patient a sense of assurance that his or her overall well-being is being considered. In some cases, physicians will not be able to agree on a patient's choice of CAM treatment and they should be able to express concerns openly (Eisenberg 1997; Lazar and O'Connor 1998). This will continue to show concern for the patient and can provide the possibility of preserving the therapeutic relationship. Further considerations have been noted by other authors regarding documentation and potential liability issues (Eisenberg 1997; Studdert et al. 1998). Nonetheless, the bottom line remains that the demand for CAM therapies does not have to result in divisive care. Instead, it can create an opportunity for ensuring comprehensive patient care and healthy patient–physician relationships.

References

Alimi Y, Di Mauro P, Fiacre E, et al: Blunt injury to the internal carotid artery at the base of the skull: six cases of venous graft restoration. J Vasc Surg 24:249–257, 1996a

Alimi Y, Tonolli I, Di Mauro P, et al: Manipulations of cervical vertebrae and trauma of the veterbral artery: report of two cases. Journal des Maladies Vasculaires 21:320–323, 1996b

Aliotta G, Pollio A: Useful plants in renal therapy according to Pliny the Elder. Am J Nephrol 14:399–411, 1994

Amor T, Todd J: Are homeopathic patients conspicuously neurotic? Psychiatr Bull 3:84–85, 1985

Anderson R, Meeker WC, Wirick BE, et al: A meta-analysis of clinical trials of spinal manipulation. J Manipulative Physiol Ther 15:181–194, 1992

Anderson W, O'Connor BB, MacGregor RR, et al: Patient use and assessment of conventional and alternative therapies for HIV infection and AIDS. AIDS 7:561–566, 1993

Astin JA: Why patients use alternative medicine: results of a national study. JAMA 279:1548–1553, 1998

Astin JA, Marie A, Pelletier KR, et al: A review of the incorporation of complementary and alternative medicine by mainstream physicians. Arch Intern Med 158:2303–2310, 1998

Balis R, Maiga A, Aboubacar A: How different are users and non-users of alternative medicine? Can J Public Health 88:159–162, 1997

Barnes J, Mills SY, Abbot NC, et al: Different standards for reporting ADRS to herbal remedies and conventional OTC medicines: face-to-face interviews with 515 users of herbal remedies. Br J Clin Pharmacol 45:496–500, 1998

Barton SE, Hawkins DA, Jadresic DM, et al: Alternative treatments for HIV infection. BMJ 298:1519–1520, 1989

Beltz SD, Doering PL: Efficacy of nutritional supplements used by athletes. Clin Pharm 12:900–908, 1993

Bendich A: Safety issues regarding the use of vitamin supplements, in Beyond Deficiency. Edited by Sauberlich HH, Machlin LJ. New York, New York Academy of Sciences, 1992, pp 300–312

Berman BM, Singh BK, Lao L, et al: Physicians' attitudes toward complementary or alternative medicine: a regional survey. J Am Board Fam Pract 8:361–366, 1995

Berman BM, Jonas W, Swyers JP: Issues in the use of complementary/alternative medical therapies for low back pain. Phys Med Rehabil Clin North Am 9:497–511, 1998a

Berman BM, Singh BB, Hartnoll SM, et al: Primary care physicians and complementary-alternative medicine: training, attitudes, and practice patterns. J Am Board Fam Pract 11:272–281, 1998b

Berman BM, Ezzo J, Hadhazy V, et al: Is acupuncture effective in the treatment of fibromyalgia? J Fam Pract 48:213–218, 1999

Blanc PD, Kuschner WG, Katz PP, et al: Use of herbal products, coffee or black tea, and over-the-counter medications as self-treatments among adults with asthma. J Allergy Clin Immunol 100:789–791, 1997

Boisset M, Fitzcharles M: Alternative medicine use by rheumatology patients in a universal health care setting. J Rheumatol 21:148-152, 1994

Brown GR, Greenwood JK: Megavitamin toxicity. Canadian Pharmacology Journal, 1987, p 79-87

Brown PJ, Carney PA: Health beliefs and alternative medicine: a qualitative study of breast cancer patients. J Cancer Educ 11:226–229, 1996

Burg MA, Hatch RL, Neims AH: Lifetime use of alternative therapy: a study of Florida residents. South Med J 91:1126–1131, 1998

But P: Need for correct identification of herbs in herbal poisoning. Lancet 341:637, 1993

But P, Chang C: Chinese herbal medicine in the treatment of asthma and allergies. Clin Rev Allergy Immunol 14:253–269, 1996

Cassileth BR: The Alternative Medicine Handbook. New York, WW Norton, 1998, pp 4–5

Cassileth BR: Complementary therapies: overview and state of the art. Cancer Nurs 22:85–90, 1999

Cassileth BR, Chapman CC: Alternative and complementary cancer therapies. Cancer 77:1026–1034, 1996a

Cassileth BR, Chapman BA: Alternative cancer medicine: a ten-year update. Cancer Invest 14:396–404, 1996b

Cassileth BR, Lusk EJ, Strouse TB, et al: Contemporary unorthodox treatments in cancer medicine: a study of patients, treatments, and practitioners. Ann Intern Med 101:105–112, 1984

Cencieros S, Brown GR: Acupuncture: a review of its history, theories, and indications. South Med J 91:1121–1125, 1998

Cherkin DC, Deyo RA, Battie M, et al: A comparison of physical therapy, chiropractic manipulation, and provision of an educational booklet for the treatment of patients with low back pain. N Engl J Med 339:1021–1029, 1998

Coleman LM, Fowler LL, Williams ME: Use of unproven therapies by people with Alzheimer's disease. J Am Geriatr Soc 43:747–750, 1995

Crocetti E, Crotti N, Feltrin A, et al: The use of complementary therapies by breast cancer patients attending conventional treatment. Eur J Cancer 34:324–328, 1998

Cronan TA, Kaplan RM, Posner L, et al: Prevalence of the use of unconventional remedies for arthritis in a metropolitan community. Arthritis Rheum 32:1604–1607, 1989

Crone CC, Wise TN: Survey of alternative medicine use among organ transplant patients. Journal of Transplant Coordination 7:123–130, 1997

Crone CC, Wise TN: Use of herbal medicines among consultation-liaison populations: a review of current information regarding risks, interactions, and efficacy. Psychosomatics 39:3–13, 1998

Davidson JR, Rampes H, Eisen M, et al: Psychiatric disorders in primary care patients receiving complementary medical treatments. Compr Psychiatry 39:16–20, 1998

Davis PA, Chang C, Hackman RM: Acupuncture in the treatment of asthma: a critical review. Allergol Immunolpathol (Madr) 26:263–271, 1998

De Matteis Tortora M: Some plants described by Pliny for the treatment of renal diseases. Am J Nephrol 14:412–417, 1994

Depierreux M, Van Damme B, Vanden Houte K, et al: Pathologic aspects of a newly described nephropathy related to prolonged use of Chinese herbs. Am J Kidney Dis 24:172–180, 1994

Dimmock S, Troughton PR, Bird HA: Factors predisposing to the resort of complementary therapies in patients with fibromyalgia. Clin Rheumatol 15:478–482, 1996

DiPalma JR, Ritchie DM: Vitamin toxicity. Annu Rev Pharmacol Toxicol 17:133–148, 1977

Donnelly WJ, Spykerboer JE, Thong YH, et al: Are patients who use alternative medicine dissatisfied with orthodox medicine? Med J Aust 142:539–541, 1985

Drivadhl CE, Miser WF: The use of alternative health care by a family practice population. J Am Fam Pract 11:193–199, 1998

Eisenberg DM: Advising patients who seek alternative medical therapies. Ann Intern Med 127:61–69, 1997

Eisenberg DM, Kessler RC, Foster C, et al: Unconventional medicine use in the United States. N Engl J Med 328:246–252, 1993

Eisenberg DM, Davis RB, Ettner SL, et al: Trends in alternative medicine use in the United States, 1990–1997. JAMA 280:1569–1575, 1998

Elder NC, Gilchrist A, Minz R: Use of alternative health care by family practice patients. Arch Fam Med 6:181–184, 1997

Eliason BC, Kruger J, Mark D, et al: Dietary supplement users: demographics, product use, and medical system interactions. J Am Board Fam Pract 10:265–271, 1997

Elion RA, Cohen C: Complementary medicine and HIV infection. Prim Care 24:905–915, 1997

Ernst E: Homeopathy revisited. Arch Intern Med 156:2162–2164, 1996

Ernst E: Life-threatening adverse reactions after acupuncture? A systematic review. Pain 71:123–126, 1997a

Ernst E: The ethics of complementary medicine. J Med Ethics 22:197–198, 1997b

Ernst E: Complementary therapies for asthma: what patients use. J Asthma 35:667–671, 1998a

Ernst E: Harmless herbs? A review of the recent literature. Am J Med 104:170–178, 1998b

Ernst E: Usage of complementary therapies in rheumatology: a systematic review. Clin Rheumatol 17:301–305, 1998c

Ernst E: Use of complementary therapies in childhood asthma. Pediatric Asthma, Allergy, and Immunology 12:29–32, 1998d

Ernst E: Complementary/alternative medicine for asthma: we do not know what we need to know. Chest 115:1–3, 1999

Ernst E, Cassileth BR: The prevalence of complementary/alternative medicine in cancer: a systematic review. Cancer 83:777–782, 1998

Eskinazi D, Hoffman FA: Progress in complementary and alternative medicine: contribution of the National Institutes of Health and the Food and Drug Administration. J Altern Complement Med 4:459–467, 1998

Fairfield KM, Eisenberg DM, Davis RB, et al: Patterns of use, expenditures, and perceived efficacy of complementary and alternative therapies in HIV-infected patients. Arch Intern Med 158:2257–2264, 1998

Fitzcharles MA, Esdaile JM: Nonphysician practitioner treatments and fibromyalgia syndrome. J Rheumatol 24:937–940, 1997

Flodin NW: Micronutrient supplements: toxicity and drug interactions. Prog Food Nutr Sci 14:277–331, 1990

Foote J, Cohen B: Medicinal herb use and the renal patient. J Renal Nutrition 8:40–42, 1998

Fulder SJ, Munro RE: Complementary medicine in the United Kingdom: patients, practitioners, and consultations. Lancet 2:542–545, 1985

Furnham A: Explaining health and illness: lay perceptions on current and future health, the causes of illness, and the nature of recovery. Soc Sci Med 39:715–725, 1994

Furnham A, Bhagrath R: A comparison of health beliefs and behaviors of clients of orthodox and complementary medicine. Br J Clin Psychol 32:237–246, 1993

Furnham A, Forey J: The attitudes, behaviors, and beliefs of patients of conventional vs. complementary (alternative) medicine. J Clin Psychol 50:458–469, 1994

Furnham A, Smith C: Choosing alternative medicine: a comparison of the beliefs of patients visiting a general practitioner and a homeopath. Soc Sci Med 26:685–689, 1988

Garewal HS, Diplock AT: How "safe" are antioxidant vitamins? Drug Saf 13:8–14, 1995

Gordon NP, Sobel DS, Tarazona EZ: Use of and interest in alternative therapies among adult primary care clinicians and adult members in a large health maintenance organization. West J Med 169:153–161, 1998

Gray RE, Fitch M, Greenberg M: A comparison of physicians and patient perspectives on unconventional cancer therapies. Psychooncology 7:445–452, 1998

Hackman RM, Stern JS, Gershwin ME: Complementary and alternative medicine and asthma. Clin Rev Allergy Immunol 14:321–337, 1996

Halbert SC: Diet and nutrition in primary care: from antioxidants to zinc. Prim Care 24:825–843, 1997

Hand R: Alternative therapies used by patients with AIDS. N Engl J Med 320:672–673, 1989

Herbert V: The antioxidant supplement myth. Am J Clin Nutr 60:157–158, 1994

Hilsden RJ, Dunn C, Patten S, et al: Information needs and seeking behaviors of patients with inflammatory bowel disease (abstract). Gastroenterology 114:A995, 1998a

Hilsden RJ, Scott CM, Verhoef MJ: Complementary medicine use by patients with inflammatory bowel disease. Am J Gastroenterol 93:697–701, 1998b

Hogan DB, Ebly EM: Complementary medicine use in a dementia clinic population. Alzheimer Dis Assoc Disord 10:63–67, 1996

Hunt JR: Position of the American Dietetic Association: vitamin and mineral supplementation. J Am Diet Assoc 96:73–77, 1996

Jacobs J, Crothers D: Who sees homeopaths? a study of patient characteristics in a homeopathic family practice. British Homeopathic Journal 80:57–58, 1991

Kaegi E: Unconventional therapies for cancer: 1. Essiac. Can Med Assoc J 158: 897–902, 1998a

Kaegi E: Unconventional therapies for cancer: 3. Iscador. Can Med Assoc J 158: 1157–1159, 1998b

Kaptchuk TJ, Eisenberg DM: Chiropractic: origins, controversies, and contributions. Arch Intern Med 158:2215–2224, 1998

Kassler WJ, Blanc P: The use of medicinal herbs by human immunodeficiency virus-infected patients. Arch Intern Med 151:2281–2288, 1991

Kleijnen J, Knipschild P, ter Riet G: Clinical trials of homeopathy. BMJ 302:316–323, 1991

Klougart N, Lebouef-Yde C, Rasmussen LR: Safety in chiropractic practice, part I: the occurrence of cerebrovascular accidents after manipulation to the neck in Denmark from 1978–1988. J Manipulative Physiol Ther 19:371–377, 1996

Kronenfeld JJ, Wasner C: The use of unorthodox therapies and marginal practitioners. Soc Sci Med 16:1119–1125, 1982

Langewitz W, Ruttimann S: The integration of alternative treatment modalities in HIV infection: the patient's perspective. J Psychosom Res 38:687–693, 1994

Lazar JS, O'Connor BB: Talking with patients about their use of alternative therapies. Prim Care 24:699–714, 1998

Lewith GT: Respiratory illness: a complementary perspective. Thorax 53:898–904, 1998

Lewith GT, Watkins AD: Unconventional therapies in asthma: an overview. Allergy 51:761–769, 1996

Linde K, Clausius N, Ramirez G, et al: Are the clinical effects of homeopathy placebo effects? A meta-analysis of placebo-controlled trials. Lancet 350:834–843, 1997

Liu JM, Chu HC, Chin YH, et al: Cross sectional study of use of alternative medicines in Chinese cancer patients. Jpn J Clin Oncol 27:37–41, 1997

MacLennan A, Wilson DH, Taylor AW: Prevalence and cost of alternative medicine in Australia. Lancet 347:569–573, 1996

Marwick C: Alterations are ahead at the OAM. JAMA 280:1553–1554, 1998

Meyers DG, Maloley PA, Weeks D: Safety of antioxidant vitamins. Arch Intern Med 156:925–935, 1996

Millar WJ: Use of alternative health care practitioners by Canadians. Can J Public Health 88:154–158, 1997

Miller DR, Anderson GT, Stark JJ, et al: Phase I/II trial of the safety and efficacy of shark cartilage in the treatment of advanced cancer. J Clin Oncol 16:3649–3655, 1998

Miller LG: Herbal medicinals: selected clinical considerations focusing on known or potential drug–herb interactions. Arch Intern Med 158:2200–2211, 1998

Montbriand MJ: An overview of alternative therapies chosen by patients with cancer. Oncol Nurs Forum 21:1547–1554, 1994

Moody GA, Eaden JA, Bhakta P, et al: The role of complementary medicine in European and Asian patients with inflammatory bowel disease. Public Health 112:269–272, 1998

Moore NG: A review of reimbursement policies for alternative and complementary medicine. Alternative Therapies 3:26–29, 1997

Moser G, Tillinger W, Sachs G, et al: Relationship between the use of unconventional therapies and disease-related concerns: a study of patients with inflammatory bowel disease. J Psychosom Res 40:503–509, 1996

Munsted K, Kirsch K, Milch W, et al: Unconventional cancer therapy: survey of patients with gynecological malignancy. Arch Gynecol Obstet 258:81–88, 1996

Nagarathna R, Nagendra HR: Yoga for bronchial asthma: a controlled study. BMJ 291:1077–1079, 1985

National Institutes of Health Consensus Development Panel on Acupuncture: NIH consensus conference: acupuncture. JAMA 280:1518–1524, 1998

Nicassio PM, Schuman C, Kim J, et al: Psychosocial factors associated with complementary treatment use in fibromyalgia. J Rheumatol 24:2008–2013, 1997

Oneschuk D, Fennell L, Hanson J, et al: The use of complementary medications by cancer patients attending an outpatient pain and symptom clinic. J Palliat Care 14:21–26, 1998

Ostrow MJ, Cornelisse PG, Heath KV, et al: Determinants of complementary therapy use in HIV-infected individuals receiving antiretroviral or anti-opportunistic agents. J Acquir Immune Defic Syndr Hum Retrovirol 15:115–120, 1997

Paramore LC: Use of alternative therapies: estimates from the 1994 Robert Wood Johnson Foundation National Access to Care Survey. J Pain Symptom Manage 13:83–89, 1997

Paulsen SM: Use of herbal products and dietary supplements by oncology patients: informed decisions? Highlights in Oncology Practice 15:94–106, 1998

Pioro-Boisset M, Esdaile JM, Fitzcharles MA: Alternative medicine use in fibromyalgia syndrome. Arthritis Care and Research 9:13–17, 1996

Resch KL, Hill S, Ernst E: Use of complementary therapies by individuals with "arthritis." Clin Rheumatol 16:391–395, 1997

Reynolds RD: Vitamin supplements: current controversies. J Am Coll Nutr 13:118–126, 1994

Risberg T, Bremnes RM, Wist E, et al: Communicating with and treating cancer patients: how does the use of non-proven therapies and patients' feeling of mental distress influence the interaction between the patient and the hospital staff. Eur J Cancer 33:883–890, 1997

Risberg T, Lund E, Wist E, et al: Cancer patients' use of nonproven therapy: a 5-year follow-up study. J Clin Oncol 16:6–12, 1998a

Risberg T, Wist E, Bremnes RM: Patients' opinions and use of non-proven therapies related to their view of cancer aetiology. Anticancer Res 18:499–505, 1998b

Senstad O, Lebouef-Yde C, Borchgrevnik CF: Side effects of chiropractic manipulation: types, frequency, discomfort, and course. Scand J Prim Health Care 14:50–53, 1996

Senstad O, Leboeuf-Yde C, Borchgrevnik C: Frequency and characteristics of side effects of spinal manipulative therapy. Spine 22:435–440, 1997

Shekelle PG, Adams AH, Chassin MR: Spinal manipulation for low-back pain. Ann Intern Med 117:590–598, 1992

Singh N, Squier C, Sivek C, et al: Determinants of nontraditional therapy use in patients with HIV infection. Arch Intern Med 156:197–201, 1996

Snyder P: The use of nonprescribed treatments by hemodialysis patient. Cult Med Psychiatry 7:57–76, 1983

Studdert DM, Eisenberg DM, Miller FH, et al: Medical malpractice implications of alternative medicine. JAMA 20:1610–1615, 1998

Sugarman J, Burk L: Physicians' ethical obligations regarding alternative medicine. JAMA 280:1623–1625, 1998

Sutherland LR, Verhoef MJ: Why do patients seek a second opinion or alternative medicine? Clin Gastroenterol 19:194–197, 1994

Thomas KJ, Carr J, Westlake L, et al: Use of non-orthodox and conventional health care in Great Britain. BMJ 302:207–210, 1991

van Ypersele de Strihou C, Vanherweghem JL: The tragic paradigm of Chinese herb nephropathy. Nephrol Dial Transplant 10:157–160, 1995

VandeCreek L, Rogers E, Lester J: Use of alternative therapies among breast cancer outpatients compared with the general population. Altern Ther Health Med 5:71–76, 1999

Vanhaelen M, Vanhaelen-Fastre R, But P, et al: Identification of aristolochic acid in Chinese herbs. Lancet 343:174, 1994

Vanherweghem JL, Depierreux M, Tielemans C, et al: Rapidly progressive interstitial renal fibrosis in young women: association with slimming regimen including Chinese herbs. Lancet 341:387–391, 1993

Vecchio PC: Attitudes to alternative medicines by rheumatology outpatient attenders. J Rheumatol 21:145–147, 1994

Verhoef MJ, Sutherland LR: Use of alternative medicine by patients attending a gastroenterology clinic. CMAJ 142:121–125, 1990

Verhoef MJ, Scott CM, Hilsden RJ: A multimethod research study on the use of complementary therapies among patients with inflammatory bowel disease. Altern Ther Health Med 4:68–71, 1998

Vickers AJ, Smith C: Analysis of the evidence profile of the effectiveness of complementary therapies in asthma: a qualitative study and systematic review. Complement Ther Med 5:202–209, 1997

Vickers AJ, Rees RW, Robin A: Advice given by health food shops: is it clinically safe? J R Coll Physicians Lond 32:426–428, 1998

Vincent C, Furnham A: Why do patients turn to complementary medicine? An empirical study. Br J Clin Psychol 35:37–48, 1996

Wetzel MS, Eisenberg DM, Kaptchuk TJ: Courses involving complementary and alternative medicine at U.S. medical schools. JAMA 280:784–787, 1998

Winterholler M, Erbguth F, Neundorfer B: The use of alternative medicine by multiple sclerosis patients: patient characteristics and patterns of use. Fortschr Neurol Psychiatr 65:555–561, 1997

Afterword

Philip R. Muskin, M.D.

Learning is always a journey. The intention of this book is to start psychiatrists and other mental health professionals on the journey toward a more complete understanding of complementary and alternative medicine (CAM). Only a small number of topics could be included in this volume; many others might have been chosen. To provide foundations for a bridge between the practice of psychiatry and the use of CAM, the "bias" here has been areas in which the experts are both physicians and practitioners of CAM. Some of what has been presented may seem dramatically different from that with which we are accustomed, but much is quite familiar. As much as possible, the original sources have been provided for those who wish to review the material on their own.

There is clearly a need for continued research to elucidate the active ingredients in herbs and to fully explore the value of acupuncture, meditative techniques, and yoga. Realistically, there will never be enough research to completely answer all of our questions. Clinical medicine always relies on the experience of practitioners to separate prospective treatments that have efficacy from those that do not. Research often proves that which we already know. Occasionally there are surprises, as when therapies we believe to have value do not hold up to the spotlight of double-blind, placebo-controlled studies. Methodologic problems pose difficulties for research into CAM therapies, perhaps with the exception of herbal products and nutrients. If we can identify the active ingredients in a natural substance, perhaps the same genius that has inspired pharmacologic research can provide information about the large number of substances that have yet to be investigated. Can those same research methodologies be expanded into the investigation of nonpharmacologic CAM therapies? Although thousands of years of practice may not "prove" the value of an alternative technique as a therapy for illness, something of significance has maintained the practice for so many years. Working with reputable practitioners of CAM therapies, we may discover the essential therapeutic elements so that they may be routinely incorporated into the treatment of patients.

The public would be better served if the government chose to control herbal and nutrient products not as dietary supplements, but as pharmaceutical products. This is the situation in Germany, where herbal products are strictly controlled and their use requires a prescription. In the United States, dietary supplements are not subjected to the rigorous clinical investigation and quality control that we expect from medications. We must recognize that alternative products are an industry worth many billions of dollars. If the products are subjected to clinical study, and do not meet the U.S. Food and Drug Administration's requirements of efficacy, the potential loss in revenue is considerable. Whether the interests of the public or the industry will prevail here will depend on which group attracts the attention and the concern of the Congress.

In the final analysis, we must distinguish the practice of medicine from the discipline of science. Dr. James S. Goodwin's comments on science and medicine provide insight in relation to an approach toward CAM and psychiatry:

> A physician is a practitioner, not a scientist. Much of the knowledge base available to physicians comes from scientific investigation. Science provides information about the average behavior of groups—groups of molecules or kidneys or human beings. The practicing physician can use that information in making decisions about the care of individual patients.
>
> Much of modern medicine seems based not on science but on scientism, a belief system in which the trappings of science—the machines, the digital readouts, the P values—acquire a legitimacy independent of their utility in addressing the actual problems at hand. Scientific dogma can be invoked to justify either undertreatment or overtreatment. Wise, responsive clinical care is something else again. (Goodwin 1999, p. 769)

We are preparing this book at the start of a new century and a new millennium. Perhaps in this new millennium, we can augment current therapies by employing science to wisely incorporate 2,000 years of CAM therapies into conventional practice.

Reference

Goodwin JS: Geriatrics and the limits of medicine (letter). N Engl J Med 341:769, 1999

Index

*Page numbers printed in **boldface** type refer to tables or figures.*

Adapton. *See* Fish extract
Addiction
    acupuncture for, 90, 213
    allostatic load and, 158
    meditation for, 154, 173, 174
    yoga for, 134
Adenosine triphosphate (ATP), 7
S-Adenosylmethionine (SAMe),
    6–17
    advantages of, 10
    for age-related memory
        impairment, 13
    for attention-deficit disorder
        with hyperactivity, 13
    biochemistry of, 7–8
    brand names of, 16
    cost of, 16
    discovery of, 8
    disorders associated with low
        cerebrospinal fluid levels
        of, 8
    dosage and administration of,
        11, 16
    drug interactions with, 14
    evidence for use in depression,
        8–11
        compared with standard
            antidepressants, 8–12,
            16–17
        postmenopausal
            depression, 9
        postpartum depression, 9
        treatment-resistant
            depression, 9, 12
    for fibromyalgia, 12
    formulations of, 8, 16
    hypomania induced by, 9
    mechanism of action of, 7
    for osteoarthritis, 7, 8, 13–14,
        16
    for other disorders, 14

    for Parkinson's disease, 8, 13
    regulation of, 7
    side effects of, 10, 13–15
    use during pregnancy and
        lactation, 15
    use in patients with serious
        medical conditions, 14–15
ADHD (attention-deficit
    disorder with hyperactivity)
    S-adenosylmethionine for, 13
    omega-3 fatty acids for, 42
Adhisiksya, **151**, **152**, 156
α-Adrenergic blockers, 33
Adrenocorticotropic hormone
    (ACTH), 89, 214
Advaityajnana, **152**
Adverse effects, 2, 207, 208
    of S-adenosylmethionine, 10,
        13–15
    of α–adrenergic blockers, 33
    of calcium supplements, 26
    of carbamazepine, 22
    deaths from, 2–3
    of finasteride, 33
    of ginkgo, 38
    of herbs, 2–3, 217, **218–218**
        herb–drug interactions, xx,
            1, 2, 47–48, 217, **220**
    of hormone replacement
        therapy, 28
    of kava, 19–20
    of licorice, 30
    of nonsteroidal anti-
        inflammatory drugs, 2, 211
    of nutritional supplements,
        225, **226–227**
    of St. John's wort, 4–5
    of valerian, 21
    of yohimbine, 35
Agency for Health Care Policy
    and Research (AHCPR), 212

Aggression, docosahexanoic acid levels and, 42
Ah Shi points, 99
Ahamkara, 116
AHCPR (Agency for Health Care Policy and Research), 212
Ahimsa, 118
AIDS. *See* Human immunodeficiency virus infection
Akasopama-samahita, **151**
ALA (α-linolenic acid), 43
Alayavijnana, **153**
Alcar. *See* Acetyl L-carnitine
Alcohol withdrawal, 14
Alcoholic liver disease, 14
Aldosterone, 25, 135
Allergies, 204, 223
Allium sativum (garlic), xx, 47, **220**
Allopathic medicine, xv–xvii, xxvi, 200
　patient dissatisfaction with, 207–209
Allostatic load, 158, 165, 167
Aloe *(Aloe vera)*, **218, 220**
Alprazolam, 20
Alternate nostril breathing, 131, 132, 136
Alternative Medicine Yellow Pages, 201
Alzheimer's disease, 28, 216
　acetyl L-carnitine for, 39
　S-adenosylmethionine and, 8, 13
　allostatic load and, 158
　docosahexanoic acid levels and, 42
　ginkgo for, 38
　phosphatidyl serine for, 41
American Botanical Council, 48, 49

γ-Aminobutyric acid (GABA) receptors
　kava and, 18
　valerian and, 21
Amitriptyline, 4, 9
Amok, 86
Analgesia, 204, 211–212
　acupuncture for, 88, 90, 213–214
　kava for, 18
　meditation for, 156, 162
　yoga for, 137–139
Analytic insight meditation, 154–155, 161
Ananda marga tantric yoga, 176
Androstenedione, 33
Anesthesia–herb reactions, xx, 47
Angelica sinensis (dong quai), **220**
　for menopausal symptoms, 30–31
Angina pectoris, 36
Anipryl. *See* Selegiline
Aniracetam, 40
Ankylosing spondylitis, 135, 139
Anorexia, 86, 225
Anticholinergic delirium, **220**
Anticonvulsant–herb interactions, 48
Antidepressants
　chromium picolinate for weight gain induced by, 47
　for diabetic patients, 15
　herb interactions with, xx, **220**
　placebo response and, xxiv
　tricyclic
　　adenosylmethionine compared with, 8–12, 16–17
　　compared with placebos, 100

Antidepressants *(continued)*
    tricyclic *(continued)*
        phosphatidyl serine for
            memory problems
            induced by, 41
        rapid eye movement sleep
            behavior disorder
            induced by, 22
        safety of long-term use of,
            10
        St. John's wort compared
            with, 3–5
Antihistamines, **220**
Antihypertensive agents, 101, **220**
Antineoplastic agents, xix
Antioxidants
    S-adenosylmethionine and, 7,
        10
    melatonin, 44
    nutritional supplements,
        224–225
Antiparkinsonian agents, **220**
Antipsychotics, **220**
Antiretroviral therapy, 223
Antispasmodic agents, **220**
Anupalambha-karuna, **153**
Anuttara yoga tantra, **152,** 168,
    176
Anuvrtti, **150**
Anxiety, 204. *See also* specific
    anxiety disorders
    acupuncture for, 89, **93**
    allostatic load and, 158
    culture and, 87
    herbs and nutrients for, 18–21
        chamomile, 20
        fish extract, 20–21
        kava, 18–20
        lemon balm, 20
        passion flower, 20
        valerian, 21

induced by
    S-adenosylmethionine, 14
induced by yohimbine, 35
meditation for, 154, 156, 162,
    175, 176
stress response and, 157
yoga for, 111, 126, 127, 131–132
Aparigraha, 118–119
Apigenin, 20
Appetite changes, premenstrual,
    24
Apramana-dhyana, **152**
Arginine, 36
Aromatase, 33, 34
Arousal state during meditation,
    168
Artemesia vulgaris (moxa), 96
Arthritis, 204, 211
    acupuncture for, 90
    S-adenosylmethionine for, 7, 8,
        13–14, 16
    dehydroepiandrosterone for,
        45
    feverfew for, 23
    glucosamine for, 228
    yoga for, 139
Aryasatya, 162
Asana, 120–121, **122**
Ascetic practices in yoga, 119
Aspirin, xviii
Asteya, 118
Asthma, 221–222
    acupuncture for, 90, 222
    yoga for, 131, 136–137, 222
Astragalus, 48
Athletic enhancement, 48
Atisha, 156
Atmagrahabandha, **150**
Atmagrahavasana, **150**
Atman, 116
ATP (adenosine triphosphate), 7

Bone density
   chromium picolinate and, 46
   dehydroepiandrosterone and,
      45
Borage oil, 48
Borderline personality disorder
   (BPD)
   dialectical behavior therapy
      for, 176
   meditation for, 156, 179
BPH. *See* Benign prostatic
   hypertrophy
Brahmacharya, 118
Braid, James, xxii
Brain, stress effects on, 161
Brain imaging studies, xxiii, 14,
   18, 165
Breast cancer, xxiv, xxv
   black cohosh and, 30
   hormone replacement therapy
      and, 28
   soy products and, 29
Breast feeding
   S-adenosylmethionine and,
      15
   chasteberry and, 27
Breathing techniques
   in process meditative
      practices, 167
   in yoga, 113, 115, 121
Bronchodilators, 221
Bruxism, induced by St. John's
   wort, 4, 6
Buckthorn, **220**
Buddhi, 116
Buddhist traditions, 78, 107, 129,
   155, **172**
Bupropion, 41
Burdock, **220**
Burns, dehydroepiandrosterone
   for, 45

Cachexia, 225
Caffeine–ephedrine combination,
   for obesity, 47
Cakra, **152**
Calcitonin gene-related peptide,
   89
Calcium, for premenstrual
   syndrome, 26
CAM. *See* Complementary and
   alternative medicine
cAMP (cyclic adenosine
   monophosphate), 17
Cancer, 204, 228–230
   breast, xxiv, xxv
      black cohosh and, 30
      hormone replacement
         therapy and, 28
      soy products and, 29
   prostate, 37
   shark cartilage for, 225, **227**
Candali, **151,** 168
Carbamazepine, 22
Carbohydrates, for premenstrual
   syndrome, 26
Catnip, **220**
Caulophyllum thalictroides (blue
   cohosh), for menopausal
   symptoms, 32
CBT. *See* Cognitive-behavioral
   therapy
Cerebral blood flow during
   meditation, 168
Cerebral laterality in meditation,
   164–165
Cerebrospinal fluid
   S-adenosylmethionine
   levels, 8
Cetana, **151**
CGI (Clinical Global Impression),
   5, 19
Chakra, 123, 130, 168

Chamomile *(Matricaria recutita),* **220**
    for anxiety, 20
Chandana, **151**
Channels in traditional Chinese medicine, 76, **77**
Chaparral *(Larrea tridentata),* **218**
Chasteberry *(Vitex agnus castus)*
    mechanism of action of, 27
    for menopausal symptoms, 31
    for premenstrual syndrome, 27
Chemotherapy agents, xix
Childhood neglect, 176
Chills, induced by yohimbine, 35
Chinese medicine. *See* Traditional Chinese medicine
Chiropractic, xxi, 200, 212–213
Choline
    for cognitive enhancement, 39–40
    for mood disorders, 18
Christian Science, xxi
Chromium picolinate, 48, 225, **227**
    for obesity, 46–47
Chromium Picolinate: Everything You Need to Know, 46
Chronic fatigue syndrome, 86
Chronic illness, 210–217
    acupuncture for, 213–214
    arthritis, low back pain, and fibromyalgia, 211–212
    chiropractic for, 212–213
    dementia, 216
    herbal medicine for, 217, **218–220**
    inflammatory bowel disease, 214–215
    renal failure, 215–216

Chrysin, 20
Cimicifuga racemosa (black cohosh), **218**
    for menopausal symptoms, 29–30
Cinta-mayi-prajna, **151**
Cirrhosis, 14
Citta, **151**
Clinical Global Impression (CGI), 5, 19
Clomipramine, 9, 10
Clonazepam, 22
Coagulation disorders, 230
    acupuncture and, 214
    induced by ginkgo, 38
Cocaine Alternative Treatments Study, 95
Coenzyme Q-10
    for cognitive enhancement, 40
    combined with acetyl L-carnitine, 39
Cognitive-behavioral therapy (CBT), 157, 159
    meditation and, 162–163, 174, 176
    yoga and, 127, 129–130
Cognitive enhancement, 38–46
    acetyl L-carnitine for, 39
    choline for, 39–40
    dehydroepiandrosterone for, 43–46
    ginkgo for, 38
    ginseng for, 40
    α-lipoic acid and coenzyme Q-10 for, 40
    melatonin for, 43–44
    nootropic compounds for, 40
    omega-3 fatty acids for, 42–43
    phosphatidyl serine for, 41
    selegiline for, 39
Cold in Yin-Yang theory, 70–71

Cortisol, 135, 159
Crataegeus laevigata; Crataegeus monogyna (hawthorn), **218, 220**
Creative inhibition, 176
Crohn's disease, 214
Crying, premenstrual, 24
Cullen, William, xxi
Culture and psychiatry, 86–88
Culture-bound syndromes, 86
Cyclic adenosine monophosphate (cAMP), 17
Cyclosporine, 48

Dampness in Yin-Yang theory, 70
Dandelion, **220**
Dass, Ram, 109
DBT (dialectical behavior therapy), 176
"De Qi," 89, 97
Defensive reactivity, meditation and, 158–159, 167, 169
Dehydroepiandrosterone (DHEA), 33, 225, **227**
  for cognitive enhancement, 43–46
  for depression, 45
  for other disorders, 45
Delirium, anticholinergic, **220**
Dementia, 216. *See also* Alzheimer's disease
  S-adenosylmethionine for, 13
  docosahexaenoic acid levels and, 42
  melatonin for insomnia in, 22
Denial, xxvi
Depression, 204
  acetyl L-carnitine for, 39
  acupuncture for, 89, **92, 93**
  S-adenosylmethionine for, 8–11
  allostatic load and, 158

culture and, 87
dehydroepiandrosterone for, 45
docosahexaenoic acid levels and, 42
induced by α-adrenergic blockers, 33
menopause and, 28
as neural plasticity disorder, 158
nutrients for, 17–18
premenstrual, 24
seasonal affective disorder, 4, 6
St. John's wort for, xxii, 3–6
in traditional Chinese medicine, 79, 83–85, **84**
yoga for, 131, 132
Desensitization, 174, 179
Desikachar, T. K. V., 142
Desipramine, 9
Devi, Indra, 109
Devotion to the Lord, in yoga, 120
Dexfenfluramine, 47
DHA (docosahexaenoic acid), 41–43
Dharana, 123
Dharani, **151**
DHEA. *See* Dehydroepiandrosterone
DHT (dihydrotestosterone), 33, 34, 45
Dhyana, **150, 151**
Diabetes
  S-adenosylmethionine versus standard antidepressants for, 15
  chromium picolinate for, 46
  ginseng for, 40
  steroid-induced, 211
  yoga for, 138–139

Diagnostic and Statistical Manual of Mental Disorders (DSM), 86, 87, 95, 131, 141

Dialectical behavior therapy (DBT), 176

Dialysis patients, 215–216

Dietary Supplement Health and Education Act of 1994, xix

Dietary supplements. See Herbs and nutrients

Digitalis purpurea (foxglove), xix, **220**

Digitalis toxicity, **220**

Digitoxin, xix

Digoxin, 48, **220**

Dihydrotestosterone (DHT), 33, 34, 45

Dimethylglycine, 8

Diuretics, 48, **220**

Dizziness
induced by α-adrenergic blockers, 33
induced by yohimbine, 35

Docosahexaenoic acid (DHA), 41–43

Dong quai (Angelica sinensis), **220**
for menopausal symptoms, 30–31

Dopamine, 25
acupuncture and, 89
S-adenosylmethionine and, 7, 14
St. John's wort and, 5
yoga and, 135

Doxazosin, 33

Drives, in yoga, 128–129

Dropsy, xix

Drug–herb interactions, xx, 1, 2, 47–48, 217, **220**

Dry mouth, induced by S-adenosylmethionine, 13

Dryasatya, **152**

Dryness in Yin-Yang theory, 70

DSM (Diagnostic and Statistical Manual of Mental Disorders), 86, 87, 95, 131, 141

Duhkha-satya, **152**

Dyana, 123

Dynorphins, 89

Dysmenorrhea, 90

Dyspnea, induced by kava, 19

Dysthymia
chromium picolinate for, 47
dehydroepiandrosterone for, 45
meditation for, 176

Dystonia, induced by valerian, 21

Dzog chen, 176

Earth in Five Phase theory, 71–73, **72, 73**

ECG (electrocardiogram) findings, 20

Echinacea purpurea, xx, 48

Ecstasy in yoga, 116, 123–124

Eczema, xix

Eddy, Mary Baker, xxi

Edema, xix

EEG (electroencephalogram) findings, 22, 137, 149, 154, 163, 166, 168, 169

Ego, in yoga, 116, 117

Eicosapentaenoic acid (EPA), 43

Ejaculatory dysfunction, induced by α-adrenergic blockers, 33

Ekagrana-samadhi, **150**

Ekayana, **153**

Eldepryl. See Selegiline

Electrocardiogram (ECG) findings, 20

Gestalt therapy, 127
Ginger, 47
Ginkgo *(Ginkgo biloba)*
　for cognitive enhancement, 38
　combined with phosphatidyl
　　serine, 41
　dosage of, 38
　drug interactions with, xx, 47,
　　220
　for sexual enhancement, 36
　side effects of, 38
Ginseng *(Panax ginseng),* 48, **218**
　for cognitive enhancement,
　　40
　drug interactions with, 47, **220**
　for sexual enhancement, 35–36
Glaucoma, 137
Glucosamine, 228
Glutathione, 7
Glycyrrhiza glabra (licorice), **218**
　drug interactions with, 48, **220**
　for menopausal symptoms,
　　30
Goodwin, James S., 242
Graham, Sylvester, xvii
The Green Pharmacy, 49
GSR (galvanic skin response),
　168
Gtong-len, **151**
gTum-mo, **151,** 168
Guided imagery, 176
Gunas, 113
Guru, **151**
Gymnema sylvestre, **220**
Gynecology clinicians, 205

Hahnemann, Samuel, xviii
Halcion. *See* Alprazolam
Hallucinations, **91**
Hamilton Anxiety Rating Scale
　(Ham-A), 19, 131

Hamilton Rating Scale for
　Depression (Ham-D), 5, 12,
　131
Hatha yoga, 109, 125, 127, 134,
　142, 153
Hawthorn *(Crataegeus laevigata;
　Crataegeus monogyna),* **218,
　220**
Headache, 204
　acupuncture for, 213
　feverfew for migraine,
　　23–24
　induced by
　　S-adenosylmethionine, 13,
　　14
　induced by α-adrenergic
　　blockers, 33
　induced by calcium
　　supplements, 26
　induced by drugs for HIV
　　infection, 223
　induced by ginkgo, 38
　induced by hormone
　　replacement therapy, 28
　induced by saw palmetto, 33
　induced by yohimbine, 35
　melatonin for cluster
　　headaches, 44
　premenstrual, 24
　yoga for, 138
Heart disease, xxvii, 7
　acupuncture and, 214
　S-adenosylmethionine and, 7,
　　14–15
　hormone replacement therapy
　　and, 28
　meditation for, 147, 154
　omega-3 fatty acids and, 43
　among postmenopausal
　　women, 28
　yoga for, 136, 140

Jing, 74, 75
Jitteriness, induced by St. John's wort, 4, 6
Jnana, **150**
Jnana yoga, 108
Jneyavarana, **152**
Joint disorders, yoga for, 135
Jois, Pattabhi, 109
Jones, Jennifer, 109
Juniper, **220**
Justice, 206

Kaivalyadhama, 108
Kalayanamitra, **151**
Kapalabhati breathing, 121, 132, 134
Karma, 108, **150,** 161
Karuna, **150**
Kashmiri Shaivite tantra, 176
Kava *(Piper methysticum),* 18–20, 230
    analgesic properties of, 18
    anticonvulsant properties of, 18
    dosage of, 18
    drug interactions with, 48, **220**
    efficacy for anxiety, 19
    mechanism of action of, 18
    side effects and toxicity of, 19–20, **218**
    as skeletal muscle relaxant, 18
Kindling, meditation and, 167–169
Klesa, **150**
Klesavarana, **153**
Klesha, 161
Klista-karma, **150**
Knee disorders, yoga for, 135
Kommission E (Germany), 3
Krishnamacharya, 109
Kriya, 119, 132, 136, 137
Kundalini yoga, 119, 120, 130, 176
Kuvalayananda, 108

Lactation
    chasteberry-induced increase of, 27
    use of *S*-adenosylmethionine during, 15
Larrea tridentata (chaparral), **218**
Latah, 86
Laxatives, herbal, 48
Laya, 120
Learned helplessness, 158
Learning
    effects of stressful versus enriched environments on, 159
    meditation and psychotherapy as methods of enriched learning, 161–170
    models of meditation, 155–157
    neural plasticity and, 159
Lectures on the Science of Life, xvii
Lemon balm *(Melissa officinalis),* for anxiety, 20
Lepidium peruvianum chacon (maca), for sexual enhancement, 37–38
Levodopa, 8, 22
LH (luteinizing hormone), 27–29, 31
Licorice *(Glycyrrhiza glabra),* **218**
    drug interactions with, 48, **220**
    for menopausal symptoms, 30
Life-threatening illness, 221–230
    asthma, 221–222
    cancer, 228–230
    HIV disease, 223–224
    homeopathy for, 222–223
    nutritional supplements for, 224–228, **226–227**
Light on Pranayama, 142
Lily-of-the-valley, 220

α-Linolenic acid (ALA), 43
α-Lipoic acid
for cognitive enhancement, 40
combined with acetyl
L-carnitine, 39
Lithium, 18
Lobelia, **220**
Loose bowels
induced by *S*-
adenosylmethionine, 13,
14
induced by drugs for HIV
infection, 223
induced by inositol, 17
induced by St. John's wort, 4
Lucid altered states, 167
Lupus erythematosus, 45
Lust, Benedict, 108
Luteinizing hormone (LH),
27–29, 31
Lycopene, 45

Ma huang *(Ephedra sinica)*, xx,
219, 222
Maca *(Lepidium peruvianum
chacon)*, for sexual
enhancement, 37–38
Mad cow disease, 41
Madhavadasaji, Paramahansa,
108
Magnesium
for asthma, 222
for premenstrual syndrome,
25
Magnetic resonance imaging
(MRI), 14, 18
Mahabharata, 107
Mahamudra, **151,** 176
Mahanispanna, **151**
Mahayana, **153,** 161
Maitri, **151**

Manas, 116, **151**
Manasayatana, **153**
Manaskara, **150**
Mandala, **151, 153,** 162, 168
Mania. *See also* Bipolar disorder
choline for, 18
culture and, 87
induced by inositol, 17
Mantra, 123, **151,** 153, 167
Mantrayana, **153**
MAOIs. *See* Monoamine oxidase
inhibitors
Marapuama *(Ptychopetalum
guyanna)*, for sexual
enhancement, 37
Marga-satya, **152**
Massage, xxi, 230
Mastamani, Yogendra, 108
Matricaria recutita (chamomile),
220
for anxiety, 20
Mayadeha, **153**
Medical ethics, 206
Medical illness, 206–210. *See also*
specific conditions
chronic, 210–217
acupuncture for, 90, 213–
214
arthritis, low back pain, and
fibromyalgia, 211–212
chiropractic for, 212–213
dementia, 216
herbal medicine for, 217,
218–220
inflammatory bowel
disease, 214–215
renal failure, 215–216
life-threatening, 221–230
asthma, 221–222
cancer, 228–230
HIV disease, 223–224

homeopathy for, 222–223
nutritional supplements for,
   224–228, **226–227**
use of *S*-adenosylmethionine
   in patients with, 14–15
yoga for, 135–139
The Medical Letter, 44, 48
Meditation, xxi, xxii, 147–180,
   200. *See also* Yoga
alliance in practice of, 177
arousal during, 168
Asian systems of, 148, 149,
   154, 171
attentional alterations in, 155,
   156, 163–164
brain imaging studies of, 165
bridge of hypnotic learning
   from meditation to
   psychotherapy, 149–157
clinical indications for, 170–171
comparison of typologies of,
   171–173, **172**
as complement to
   psychopharmacology, 179
course and outcome of, 178
definition of, 147
early research on, 149–154
evidence for use as stress-
   reduction technique, 148
hypnosis and, 148, 154,
   156–157, 173, 176, 180
learning model of, 155–157
in medicine, neuroscience, and
   psychiatry, 147–149, 156,
   173–176
anxiety, 154, 156, 162, 175,
   176
indications for advance
   process practices, 176
substance abuse, 154, 173,
   174

therapeutic alliance and,
   177
mindfulness, 154–155,
   161–165, 171
analytic insight and, 165
cerebral laterality and,
   164–165
physiology of, 163
relation to free association
   and cognitive therapy,
   162–163, 171–173
relationship to rest, 163
as part of multicomponent
   lifestyle therapies, 178
patient satisfaction with, 178
placebo effect and, 149
problems in research on, 149
psychotherapy and, 148,
   171–173, 179–180
relaxed alertness for, 155, 163,
   165, 167, 168
research and teaching uses of,
   170
Sanskrit terms and English
   equivalents related to,
   150–153
stages of integrated
   concentrative and analytic
   meditation, **160,** 161–162
individual meditative
   practices, 162–165
process meditative
   practices, 167–170
social meditative practices,
   165–167
stress, learning, and the brain,
   157–161
transcendental, 109, 153–154,
   162, 164, 171
in yoga, 109, 112, 123, 131
Zazen, 166, 168, 176

MEDLINE, 109
Megavitamin therapy, 225
Melatonin, **227**
  antioxidant properties of, 44
  for cluster headaches, 44
  for cognitive enhancement,
    43–44
  dosage of, 44
  for insomnia, 21–23, 44
Melissa officinalis (lemon balm),
  for anxiety, 20
Memory impairment,
  age-associated (AAMI), 38,
    216
  acetyl L-carnitine for, 39
  S-adenosylmethionine for, 13
  choline for, 39–40
  dehydroepiandrosterone for,
    43–46
  ginkgo for, 38
  ginseng for, 40
  α-lipoic acid and coenzyme
    Q-10 for, 40
  melatonin for, 43–44
  menopause and, 28
  nootropic compounds for, 40
  omega-3 fatty acids for, 42–43
  phosphatidyl serine for, 41
Menopause, female, 27–29
  clinical features of, 28
  depression and, 9
  health status and, 27–28
  herbs and nutrients for, 29–32
    black cohosh, 29–30
    blue cohosh, 32
    chasteberry, 31
    dong quai, 30–31
    hops, 31–32
    kava for anxiety, 19
    licorice, 30
    maca, 37

red clover, 29
  soy products, 29
  hormone replacement therapy
    and, 28–29
  number of women
    experiencing, 27
  yoga for, 134
Menopause, male. *See* Prostatic
  enlargement
Menstrual irregularities. *See also*
  Premenstrual syndrome
  feverfew for, 23
  during menopause, 28
Mental illness. *See also* specific
  disorders
  acupuncture for, **91–93,** 95–97
  meditation for, 156, 173–176
  among patients using
    complementary and
    alternative therapies,
    209–210
  yoga for, 130–134, 141
Mesmerism, xxi, xxii. *See also*
  Hypnosis
Metal in Five Phase theory,
  71–73, **72, 73**
Methadone treatment, 134
Methamphetamine, 14
Methionine, 89
Methylphenidate, 13
Metta, **151**
Migraine, feverfew for, 23–24
Miller, J. J., 131
Mind-body therapies, 147, 148,
  154, 157–159. *See also*
  Meditation; Yoga
Mind Cure, xxi
Mindfulness meditation,
  154–155, 161–165, 171. *See
  also* Meditation
  analytic insight and, 165

attentional alterations in, 163–164

cerebral laterality and, 164–165

physiology of, 163

relation to free association and cognitive therapy, 162, 171–173

relationship to rest, 163

relaxed alertness for, 155, 163, 165, 167

Minerals, for premenstrual syndrome, 25

Mini-Mental State Exam, 13

Minnesota Multiphasic Personality Inventory, 127

Mistletoe *(Viscum album)*, **219**

Mobility Index–Accompanied, 131

Monoamine oxidase inhibitors (MAOIs), 11

S-adenosylmethionine and, 14

St. John's wort and, 4, 48

Mood disorders. *See also* Bipolar disorder; Depression; Mania

S-adenosylmethionine for, 6–17

chromium picolinate for, 47

dehydroepiandrosterone for, 45

menopause and, 28

nutrients for, 17–18

premenstrual, 24

St. John's wort for, xxii, 3–6

stress response and, 157

Moxa *(Artemesia vulgaris)*, 96

MRI (magnetic resonance imaging), 14, 18

Multiple personality disorder, 86

Muscle relaxation, kava for, 18

MuTong, xix–xx

Myoclonus, induced by St. John's wort, 6

Nadi, **152,** 168

National Cancer Institute (NCI), 228, 229

National Center for Complementary and Alternative Medicine (NCCAM), 203–204, 228

National Institutes of Health (NIH)

Consensus Statement on Acupuncture, 90, 213

initiative on mind-body medicine, 178, 180

Office of Alternative Medicine, 109, 200, 203, 211

Native American practices, 200

Natural Medicines Comprehensive Database, 1, 49

Natural-product drugs, xviii–xix. *See also* Herbs and nutrients

Natural Product Research Consultants, 49

Naturopathy, xxi, 200

Nausea and vomiting

acupuncture for, 90, 213

herbal teas for, 230

induced by S-adenosylmethionine, 13

induced by calcium supplements, 26

induced by drugs for HIV infection, 223

induced by ginkgo, 38

induced by St. John's wort, 4

induced by yohimbine, 35

Phosphatidyl choline, 39
Phosphatidyl serine (Ptd Ser), for
  cognitive enhancement,
  41, 42
Physician training in
  complementary and
  alternative medicine, 205–206
  herbs and nutrients, 48–49
Physicians' attitudes about
  complementary and
  alternative medicine, xv,
  205–206, 231
Phytolacca americana (poke root),
  219
Pinella, 222
Piper methysticum. See Kava
Piracetam, 40
Placebo effect, xxiii–xxiv
  acupuncture research and,
    99–100
  meditation research and,
    149
Platelet aggregation inhibitors,
  220
PMS. *See* Premenstrual
  syndrome
PMS Escape, 26
Pneumothorax, acupuncture-
  induced, 90, 94, 214
Po (Corporeal Soul), 79–81
Poke root *(Phytolacca americana)*,
  219
Positron-emission tomography
  (PET), xxiii
Posttraumatic stress disorder
  (PTSD)
  allostatic load and, 158
  yoga for, 133
Postures in yoga, 120–121, **122**
Prabhasvara, **153**
Prabhasvara-jnana, **151**

Prajna, **151,** 156
Prajna-adhisiksya, **152**
Prajnaparamita, **153**
Prakriti, 113
Pramiracetam, 40
Prana, xxi, 121, **152,** 168
Pranayama, 113, 115, 121
Pranic episodes, yoga and, 135
Prasrabdhi, **152,** 168
Pratisarana, **152**
Pratityasamutpada, **152**
Pratyahara, 113, 115, 121–123
Pratyaksa, **152**
Pregnancy
  acupuncture and, 214
  S-adenosylmethionine and, 15
  yoga during, 125, 135
Premenstrual syndrome (PMS)
  definition of, 24
  herbs and nutrients for, 24–27
    B vitamins and minerals,
      25–26
    calcium, 26
    carbohydrates, 26
    chasteberry, 27
    evening primrose oil, 24–25
    magnesium, 25
    tryptophan, 26–27
  premenstrual dysphoric
    disorder, 24, 26, 134
  yoga for, 134
Prevention of illness
  nutritional supplements for,
    225
  yoga and, 124–126
Primary care physicians, 205
Process meditative practices,
  167–170
Producing and Controlling
  cycles in Five Phase theory,
  71–73, **73**

Raga-dharma, **152**
Raja yoga, 108, 131, 162, 176
Rajas, 113
Rapid eye movement (REM)
sleep, meditation and,
167–169
Rapid eye movement (REM)
sleep behavior disorder, 22
Rdzogs-chen, **151**
Reasons for use of
complementary and
alternative medicine,
207–209, **208**
Red clover *(Trifolium pratense)*,
for menopausal symptoms,
29
5-α-Reductase, 33, 34, 45
Refraction problems, yoga for,
137
Regulation of herbal and nutrient
products, xix, 3, 217, 242
S-adenosylmethionine, 7
Reiki johrei, xxii
Relaxation response, xxii, 115,
131, 148
Relaxed alertness for meditation,
155, 163, 165, 167, 168
REM. *See* Rapid eye movement
sleep
Renal failure, 215–216, xix
Restlessness, premenstrual, 24
Retinal detachment, 137
Rheumatoid arthritis, 211
dehydroepiandrosterone for,
45
yoga for, 139
Rhinitis, induced by
α-adrenergic blockers, 33
Riboflavin (vitamin B$_2$), for mood
disorders, 17
Rig-Veda, 107

Robert Wood Johnson
Foundation National Access
to Care Survey, 204–205
Rupa-skandha, **150**
Rupra, **150**
Ryan, Robert, 109

Sabal *(Sabal serrulata)*, for benign
prostatic hypertrophy, 33
Safety
of acupuncture, 90, 94
of botanical products, xix–xx,
2–3
of long-term antidepressants,
10
Sahaja-sukha, **152**
Sahaja yoga, 176
Sahrdaya, **153**
Salicin, xviii
Samadhi, 116, 123–124, **150,** 154
Samadhi-adhisiksya, **152**
Samapatti, **150**
Samatha, **150**
Samatha-bhavana, **152**
SAMe. *See*
S-Adenosylmethionine
Samjna, **150**
Samjna-skandha, **150**
Samprajanya, **150**
Samskara, **150**
Samskara-skandha, **150**
Samudaya-satya, **152**
Sandoz Clinical Assessment
Geriatric Scale, 13
Sanskrit terms, **150–153**
Sarira, **150**
Sastr, **153**
Sat-cit-ananda, **152**
Satchidananda, Yogi Swami, 136
Sati, **151,** 154
Sattva, 113

Siddha yoga, 176
Siddhis, 119
Side effects. *See* Adverse effects
Sila-adhisiksya, **152**
Sildenafil, 35
Skeletal muscle relaxation, kava for, 18
Skin infection, acupuncture and, 214
Skin rash
  induced by ginkgo, 38
  induced by kava, 19
  phototoxic, induced by St. John's wort, 4
Skullcap, 31, **220**
Sleep disturbance. *See* Insomnia
Smrti, **151,** 154
Smuts, J. C., xxii
Social meditative practices, 165–167
Somatoform disorders, 87–88, 101–102
Soy products, 45
  for menopausal symptoms, 29
Sparsa, **152**
Spinal manipulation, xxi, 212–213
Spiritual Axis, 80
Spironolactone, 48
Squill, **220**
Srngaranuragana, **153**
Sruta-mayi-prajna, **151**
SSRIs. *See* Selective serotonin reuptake inhibitors
St. John's wort *(Hypericum perforatum),* 3–6
  active components and response to, 4–5
  antibacterial properties of, xxiii

combined with valerian, 4
cost of, 6
dosage of, 5–6
drug interactions with, xx, 4, 47–48
effectiveness of, 6, 204
  compared with standard antidepressants, xxii, 3–5
mechanism of action of, 5
problems in previous research on, 6
quality and standardization of, 6
for seasonal affective disorder, 4, 6
side effects of, 4–6
time for response to, 6
Stabilium. *See* Fish extract
Stimulants, rapid eye movement sleep behavior disorder induced by, 22
Stinging nettle *(Urtica dioica),* for benign prostatic hypertrophy, 34
Stone, Edmund, xviii
Stress, 157–159
  allostasis and, 158
  effects on brain, 161
  learning and, 159
  sequence of response to, 157
Stress-hardiness, 155, 162
Stress reduction
  meditation for, 147–180
  yoga for, 107–142
Stroke, 7, 40
  acupuncture and, 213
  omega-3 fatty acids and, 43
Structured Clinical Interview for DSM-III, 210
Study in yoga, 119